The Rise of the Regulatory State in the Chinese Health-care System

EAI Series on East Asia

ISSN: 2529-718X

Series Editors: WANG Gungwu
(East Asian Institute, National University of Singapore)

ZHENG Yongnian
(East Asian Institute, National University of Singapore)

About the Series

EAI Series on East Asia was initiated by the East Asian Institute (EAI) (http://www.eai.nus.edu.sg). EAI was set up in April 1997 as an autonomous research organisation under a statute of the National University of Singapore. The analyses in this series are by scholars who have spent years researching on their areas of interest in East Asia, primarily, China, Japan and South Korea, and in the realms of politics, economy, society and international relations.

Published:

The Rise of the Regulatory State in the Chinese Health-care System
by QIAN Jiwei

EAI Series on
East Asia

The Rise of the Regulatory State in the Chinese Health-care System

QIAN Jiwei

East Asian Institute
National University of Singapore
Singapore

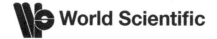

World Scientific

EW JERSEY · LONDON · SINGAPORE · BEIJING · SHANGHAI · HONG KONG · TAIPEI · CHENNAI · TOKYO

Published by

World Scientific Publishing Co. Pte. Ltd.

5 Toh Tuck Link, Singapore 596224

USA office: 27 Warren Street, Suite 401-402, Hackensack, NJ 07601

UK office: 57 Shelton Street, Covent Garden, London WC2H 9HE

Library of Congress Cataloging-in-Publication Data
Names: Qian, Jiwei, 1976–   author.
Title: The rise of the regulatory state in the Chinese health-care system / by QIAN Jiwei.
Description: New Jersey : World Scientific, [2017] | Series: EAI series on East Asia |
    Includes bibliographical references.
Identifiers: LCCN 2017001713 | ISBN 9789813207202
Subjects: | MESH: Legislation as Topic | Delivery of Health Care--
    legislation & jurisprudence | China
Classification: LCC RA395.C53 | NLM W 32.5 JC6 | DDC 362.10951--dc23
LC record available at https://lccn.loc.gov/2017001713

British Library Cataloguing-in-Publication Data
A catalogue record for this book is available from the British Library.

Desk Editor: Dong Lixi

Typeset by Stallion Press
Email: enquiries@stallionpress.com

Printed in Singapore

Contents

About the Author

Dr QIAN Jiwei is research fellow at the East Asian Institute, National University of Singapore. He obtained his BSc in computer science from Fudan University, China and PhD degree in Economics from the National University of Singapore. His research on Chinese health and social policy has been published in journals such as *The China Quarterly, Health Economics, Policy and Law, Journal of Mental Health Policy and Economics, Public Administration and Development, Public Organization Review* and *Singapore Economic Review*. His recent book is *Health Policy Reform in China: A Comparative Perspective*, co-authored with Professor Åke Blomqvist (World Scientific, 2014). His current research interests include health economics, political economy and development economics.

Abbreviations

AML:	Anti-monopoly Law
AUCL:	Anti-unfair Competition Law
BHI:	Basic Health Insurance for Urban Employees
CDC:	Chinese Centre for Disease Control and Prevention
CDE:	Centre for Drug Evaluation
CFDA:	China Food and Drug Administration
CMS:	Cooperative Medical Scheme
CNTC:	China National Tobacco Corporation
DRC:	Development and Research Centre
DRG:	Diagnosis Related Group
FCTC:	Framework Convention on Tobacco Control
FDA:	US Food and Drug Administration
FYP:	Five-Year Programme
GDP:	Gross Domestic Product
GIS:	Government Insurance Scheme
LIS:	Labour Insurance Scheme
M&A:	Mergers and Acquisitions
MIIT:	Ministry of Industry and Information Technology
MOFCOM:	Ministry of Commerce
NCMS:	New Cooperative Medical Scheme
NDRC:	National Development and Reform Commission
NEMS:	National Essential Medicine System
NOTC:	National Office of Tobacco Control

OECD: Organisation for Economic Co-operation and
           Development
SAIC: State Administration for Industry and Commerce
SOE: State-Owned Enterprises
STMA: State Tobacco Monopoly Administration
URI: Urban Resident Basic Medical Insurance
WHO: World Health Organisation

Chapter 1

Introduction

With a rapidly ageing population, the health-care system has become increasingly important in China. Health expenditure amounted to over RMB4 trillion in 2015, or 6% of gross domestic product (GDP),[1] compared to about 4% in 1997. The share of health expenditure in GDP is expected to reach 8.4% by 2030.[2] The government has also spent a huge sum of budget on health care. In 2015, government health budget amounted to over RMB1.2 trillion, accounting for about 7.12% of total fiscal expenditure compared to 4.4% in 2008. Between 2009 and 2015, total government expenditure on health reached RMB5.9 trillion, compared to RMB1.4 trillion between 1999 and 2008.[3]

Besides spending directly on health care, the government plays another important role in the health-care system as the regulator. Notably, since the 2000s, a number of regulations in social health insurance, health service quality, pharmaceutical sector, public health, antitrust and other regulations have been implemented. New regulatory agencies have been established and existing regulatory agencies have been granted more

---

[1] *Statistical Communiqué on Health and Family Planning Development in China, 2015*; see <http://www.nhfpc.gov.cn/guihuaxxs/s10748/201607/da7575d64fa04670b5f 375c87b6229b0.shtml> (accessed 24 July 2016).

[2] Ma Jun, et al., *Research on National Balance Sheet in China*, Beijing, Social Science Academic Press, 2012.

[3] *China Health Statistical Yearbook*, various years, and *Statistical Communiqué on Health and Family Planning Development in China, 2015*.

authority. For example, China Food and Drug Administration (CFDA) was promoted from a vice-ministerial to ministerial level agency in 2013. Local agencies of CFDA have been established in all provinces, in over 70% of cities and 30% of counties.[4] Regulatory reforms in the arena of public health have also been initiated, particularly at the local level. For example, in June 2015, Beijing's smoke-free regulations, the country's strictest tobacco control law, took effect, mandating all indoor and many outdoor public spaces in Beijing 100% smoke-free.[5]

Why are Regulations Necessary for the Health-care System?

Regulation refers to "rules developed and enforced by administrative agencies".[6] More specifically, regulation can be "government actions to control price, sales and production decisions of firms in the 'public interest'".[7] In the literature of comparative economics, marketisation in a transitional economy such as China's goes hand in hand with the expansion of rule-based legal institutions.[8] Regulation together with litigation can be used to correct market failures such as externalities and asymmetric information in the health-care system.[9]

---

[4] <http://news.163.com/16/0229/15/BH0JJFRB00014JB6.html> (accessed 5 May 2016).

[5] World Health Organisation, *Smoke-free Policies in China: Evidence of effectiveness and implications for action*, 2015.

[6] Daniel Kessler (ed), *Regulation Versus Litigation: Perspectives from economics and law*, Chicago, University of Chicago Press, 2011.

[7] E G Furubotn and R Richter, *Institutions and Economic Theory: The contribution of the new institutional economics*, Ann Arbor, University of Michigan Press, 2005, p. 273.

[8] Benjamin Liebman, "A Return to Populist Legality, Historical Legacies and Legal Reform", in S Heilmann and E Perry, (eds), *Mao's Invisible Hand*. Cambridge, MA, Harvard University Press, 2011. A recent discussion about the roles of formal and informal institutions in contemporary China could be found in a discussion in Chapter 1 of Lu Jie, *Varieties of Governance in China: Migration and institutional change in Chinese villages*, Oxford University Press, 2014.

[9] See a recent interesting discussion in the US context, T C Leonard, *Illiberal Reformers: Race, Eugenics, and American Economics in the Progressive Era*, Princeton University Press, 2016.

Market failures are prevalent in the health-care system in general.[10] Two types of market failure are highlighted here. First, information is asymmetric between patients and doctors, and between insurers and hospitals. For example, since patients and insurers do not have medical professional training, the quality of health-care service is not known and even observable for them, and the effects of pharmaceutical products are not fully understood by patients. Second, externalities for many public health issues are aplenty. For example, the social costs of smoking are much higher than the private costs of smoking as many people suffer from second-hand smoke.

Regulations are very useful for addressing market failures in the health-care sector.[11] First, regulations can be considered as a mechanism to internalise the externality so as to equalise private and social costs. For example, regulations to ban second-hand smoke can reduce the externality. Second, compared to litigation, the cost of the enforcement of regulations can be lower since regulations require agents such as doctors or pharmaceutical producers to fulfil certain quality requirement ex ante and service providers will be punished if those quality requirements for health-care services are not fulfilled properly. These ex ante requirements are expected to be easier to be verified compared to ex post evidences required for litigation.[12]

Third, regulations change the expectation as well as behaviour of agents in the health-care system when there is asymmetric information. Coordination among agents will be more effective. Fourth, the quality of health-care services and pharmaceutical products is expected to be able to reach a threshold level with regulations, even when patients do

---

[10] Qian Jiwei and Åke Blomqvist, *Health Policy Reform in China: A comparative perspective*, Singapore, World Scientific, 2014.

[11] Richard Posner, "Regulation (Agencies) Verses Litigation (Courts)", in D P Kessler, (ed.), *Regulation Versus Litigation: Perspectives from Economics and Law*, 2011.

[12] Edward Glaeser and Andrei Shleifer, "The Rise of the Regulatory State", *Journal of Economic Literature*, vol. 41, no. 2, 2003, pp. 401–442. See also Patricia Danzon, "The Economics of the Biopharmaceutical Industry" in *The Oxford Handbook of Health Economics*, Oxford University Press, 2011, for a similar comparison between regulation and Tort liability on the uses of pharmaceutical products.

not know the quality of services. Further, in principle, a rapid development of the private sector in the health-care system could be expected as the quality of services and products provided by the private sector has to meet the requirements stipulated in the regulations.

Literature on regulation

From the recent theoretical and empirical research, state capacity, which is defined as an "institutional capability to carry out various policies that deliver benefits and services to households and firms"[13] is pivotal to both economic and social development.[14] In particular, the government as one of the most important market-supporting institutions to regulate market is essential for achieving a more efficient allocation of resources. Financial and human capital resources of the government regulatory agencies are critical for implementing regulations. A regulatory state, in this case, depends on the government capacity to implement and enforce regulations.

However, there is also an important tradition in law and economics as well as "public choice" in which the commitment of government officials to public interests is under question. In this literature, government officials are expected to be self-interested and regulators are subject to "capture" by various interests groups.[15] Here, "capture" refers to the situation in which regulators represent the interests of the regulated. Even the federal judges in the United States may make decisions on the basis of their own preferences and interests.[16] In this case, to build up a

---

[13] Timothy Besley and Torsten Persson, *Pillars of Prosperity: The political economics of development clusters*, Princeton, Princeton University Press, 2011.

[14] See Timothy Besley and Torsten Persson, *Pillars of Prosperity* and Angus Deaton, *The Great Escape: Health, wealth, and the origins of inequality*, Princeton Jersey, Princeton University Press, 2013.

[15] Ernesto Dal Bó, "Regulatory Capture: A review", *Oxford Review of Economic Policy*, vol. 22, no. 2, 2006, pp. 203–225.

[16] Epstein Lee, William Landes and Richard Posner, *The Behavior of Federal Judges: A theoretical and empirical study of rational choice*, Cambridge, Harvard University Press, 2013.

regulatory state, incentives of the regulators must be taken into account.

Importantly, institutional arrangements for policy implementation and design are also argued to be relevant by some scholars.[17] In particular, the conceptual framework of "Fragmented Authoritarianism" has been used to understand the ineffectiveness of policymaking in China.[18] According to this framework, the fragmentation of the decision-making authority has led to a situation where interests and information become parochial. In consequence, policymaking and implementation, particularly with regard to economic policy implementation, was not very effective.[19] Recent research has shown the relevance of "Fragmented Authoritarianism" in social policy implementation in China.[20] Some peculiarities in policymaking such as logrolling have also been observed in social policymaking in China.[21] Further, in the process of transition to the market economy, regulations may also be considered as a substitute for the informal institutional arrangements in contract enforcement and dispute resolution.[22]

---

[17] For example, see Qian Jiwei "Improving Policy Design and Capacity from Local Experiments: Equalization of public service in China's urban-rural integration pilot", *Public Administration and Development*, vol. 37, no. 3, 2017, pp. 51–64.

[18] Kenneth Lieberthal and Michel Oksenberg, *Policy Making in China: Leaders, structures and processes*, Princeton, Princeton University Press, 1988.

[19] Kenneth Lieberthal, "Introduction: The 'Fragmented Authoritarianism' Model and Its Limitations", in Kenneth Lieberthal and David Lampton (eds), *Bureaucracy, Politics, and Decision Making in Post-Mao China*, Berkeley, CA, University of California Press, 1992.

[20] For example, see Qian Jiwei and Mok Ka-Ho, "Dual Decentralization and 'Fragmented Authoritarianism' in Governance: Crowding out expansion of social programmes in China", *Public Administration and Development*, vol. 36, no. 3, 2016, pp. 185–197.

[21] Mario Gilli, Li Yuan and Qian Jiwei, "Logrolling under Fragmented Authoritarianism: Theory and evidence from China", Working paper no. 333, University of Milano-Bicocca, Department of Economics, 2016.

[22] For example, see a recent study by Scott E Masten and Jens Prüfer, "On the Evolution of Collective Enforcement Institutions: Communities and courts", *Journal of Legal Studies*, vol. 43, no. 2, 2014, pp. 359–400.

Arguments of this Book

In this book, the recent development of the regulatory system in different policy areas of the Chinese health-care system will be discussed. This book will review policy development in the area of regulatory reform after a number of regulatory initiatives have been launched and several regulatory agencies established since the 2000s.

This book also highlights some important constraints in the development of the regulatory state. First, the author argues that the low capacity of regulatory agencies in both the central and local governments certainly is one major constraint. For example, there has been a shortage of manpower at the CFDA. Compared to the over 3,000 employees who work on the approval of new drugs in the Food and Drug Administration (FDA) in the United States, there are only 89 people performing the same task in the CFDA and with a queue of over 18,000 applications by the end of 2014.[23] At the local level, the shortage of resources is even more striking. For example, in Chongqing, a city with over 30 million people, the number of local CFDA staff was 22 in 2014.[24]

Second, in many cases, the incentives imposed by the regulators are not compatible with the development of the regulatory state. For example, the annual revenue of the pharmaceutical industry has reached RMB2.6 trillion in 2015 and is expected to hit RMB3 trillion in 2016.[25] For many provinces, the tax revenue from the pharmaceutical industry is significant for local fiscal revenue. Local protectionist behaviours in the pharmaceutical industry have been observed in the

---

[23] Elias Mossialos, Ge Yanfeng, Hu Jia, et al., *Pharmaceutical Policy in China, Challenges and Opportunities for Reform*, London School of Economics and Development Research Centre of the State Council of China, 2016.

[24] China National Radio, "Shiyaojianguan mianlin nanti, jiceng renshou yanzhong buzu" [Difficulties in drug regulations reforms, serious lack of local manpower], 5 October 2014, <http://china.cnr.cn/xwwgf/201410/t20141005_516549576.shtml> (accessed 24 July 2016).

[25] Guanmin web, 30 October 2015, <http://yp.gmw.cn/2015-10/30/content_17546303.htm> and <http://www.lwzb.gov.cn/pub/gjtjlwzb/sjyfx/201605/t20160525_2792.html> (accessed 22 December 2016).

government procurement process as well as other areas of regulatory policy enforcement.[26] In this case, regulation enforcement may be undermined by local protectionism. Another example is related to medical malpractice dispute resolution. For many local governments, social stability may still be one of the highly prioritised policy targets. Protesters involved in disputes concerning medical malpractices have the potential to negatively impact on the local performance on social stability.[27] Local governments largely prefer to employ more flexible dispute resolution mechanisms to reach a quick settlement with patients compared to enforcing malpractice dispute regulations.

Third and importantly, institutional arrangements are very relevant to the emergence of the regulatory state in China. The institutional structure of regulatory agencies is usually fragmented,[28] both horizontally and vertically. For example, CFDA is not the only regulator for the pharmaceutical sector. The National Development and Reform Commission (NDRC), State Ministry Administration of Industry and Commerce, as well as National Health and Family Planning Commission are also involved in regulating the pharmaceutical sector. Different regulatory agencies have different objectives; in the multiple dimensions of regulatory objectives, the enforcement in those dimensions with a lower priority may not be very effective. In a fragmented

---

[26] *Medicine Economic Reporter* [*Yiyao Jingyi Bao*], 11 November 2015, <http://www.yyjjb.com/html/2015-11/11/content_231653.htm> (accessed 24 July 2016). See a recent empirical study on local protectionism in the enforcement of advertising regulation for pharmaceutical industry by Markus Eberhardt, Wang Zheng and Yu Zhihong, "From One to Many Central Plans: Drug advertising inspections and intra-national protectionism in China", *Journal of Comparative Economics*, vol. 44, Issue 3, 2016, pp. 608–622.

[27] Benjamin Liebman, "Malpractice Mobs: Medical dispute resolution in China", *Columbia Law Review*, vol. 113, 2013, pp. 181–264.

[28] See a similar argument in the context of regulating state-owned enterprises in China in Margaret Pearson, "State-Owned Business and Party-State Regulation in China's Modern Political Economy", in *State Capitalism, Institutional Adaptation, and the Chinese Miracle*, Barry Naughton and Kellee Tsai (eds), Cambridge, Cambridge University Press, 2015.

regulatory system, blame-shifting and other opportunistic behaviours may be observed among the regulatory agencies.[29]

Many regulatory agencies have also decentralised institutional arrangements at the local level. The regulators who interact with firms and hospitals are usually from regulatory agencies at the county/city level or even lower. Such a decentralised institutional structure may undermine the regulatory capacity since the economies of scale in professional expertise and other aspects are not exploited fully.[30]

Interestingly, various institutional arrangements have been employed to address both capacity and institutional constraints of regulatory agencies. One example is to hold regular joint conferences (*Lianxi Huiyi*) on regulation in the pharmaceutical sector among relevant regulators and other stakeholders.[31] This solution improves the communications among regulatory agencies. Another example is to initiate small leading groups on implementing tobacco control policies. A small leading group consists of representatives from various ministries/regulatory agencies and a coordinator will set the policy agenda. Small leading groups can also be interpreted as a top-down solution to solve the coordination issues. Recently, to address the issue of policy ineffectiveness as a result of fragmented departmental interests, a guideline from the State Council has been released to mandate that all ministries must endorse documents within two working days of discussion and reaching a consensus at the executive meetings of the State Council.[32]

Similarly, a performance evaluation system has been applied to address the incentives of local officials. Under this performance evaluation system, appointment, promotion and demotion of local

---

[29] Tam Waikeung and Yang Dali, "Food Safety and the Development of Regulatory Institutions in China", *Asian Perspective*, vol. 29, no. 4, 2005, pp. 5–36.

[30] A similar argument in the context of tax management in China can be found in Cui Wei, "Administrative Decentralization and Tax Compliance: A transactional cost perspective", *University of Toronto Law Journal*, vol. 65, no. 3, 2015, pp. 186–238.

[31] An example of this institution is discussed in Gilli Mario, Li Yuan and Qian Jiwei, *Logrolling under Fragmented Authoritarianism: Theory and evidence from China*.

[32] Notice of the State Council, no. 31, 2015, <http://www.gov.cn/zhengce/content/2015-04/29/content_9679.htm> (accessed 25 July 2016).

bureaucrats is decided according to whether they have fulfilled the upper level government's requirements for various policy targets.[33] However, these institutional responses to the incentive and institutional structure may also have unintended consequences. For example, local officials may direct most of their efforts and resources to performance indexes which are more measurable and more rewarding and at the expense of other performance indexes.[34]

By reviewing regulatory initiatives in different areas in the health-care system, this book attempts to connect recent academic research in economics and political science with policy development in the Chinese health-care system. While there are a small number of studies on the regulations in the Chinese health-care system,[35] this book contributes to the literature in three areas. First, while more regulations have been passed, by reviewing recent cases in the Chinese health-care system, this study supports the literature that the capacity and incentives of the regulatory agencies matter in the implementation and enforcement of the regulations. Second, this study underlines some institutional arrangements in China which are particularly important to configuring the capacity and incentives of the regulatory system.

---

[33] Li Hongbin and Zhou Lian, "Political Turnover and Economic Performance: The incentive role of personnel control in China", *Journal of Public Economics*, vol. 89, no. 9–10, 2005, pp. 1743–1762 and Victor Shih, et al., "Getting Ahead in the Communist Party: Explaining the advancement of Central Committee members in China", *American Political Science Review*, vol. 106, no. 1, 2012, pp. 166–187.

[34] Qian Jiwei and Mok Ka-Ho, "Dual Decentralization and 'Fragmented Authoritarianism' in Governance".

[35] For example, Fang Jing. "The Chinese Health Care Regulatory Institutions in an Era of Transition", *Social Science and Medicine*, vol. 66, no. 4, 2008, pp. 952–962; Yang Dali, "Regulatory Learning and its Discontents in China: Promise and tragedy at the State Food and Drug Administration", in *Regulation in Asia: Pushing Back on Globalization*, John Gillespie and Randall Peerenboom, (eds), London and New York, Routledge, 2009, pp. 115–134. Yang Tuan and Shi Yuxiao. "Governance and Regulation: An alternative to the stalemate in health reform program in China", *Social Sciences in China*, vol. 27, 2006, pp. 117–133. Huang Yanzhong. *Governing Health in Contemporary China*, Abingdon and New York, Routledge, 2013.

Third, by focusing on the case of China, this book also contributes to the literature by laying out institutional reasons for the ineffectiveness of regulatory reforms in China.

There are two possible explanations to these institutional constraints of regulatory reforms. One explanation is from the macro level. Regulatory reforms are usually second best and policymakers have to trade-off between various policy targets at times. Occasionally, institutional arrangements under these reforms also have unintended consequences. For example, the performance evaluation system encourages officials to be accountable to upper level governments but local officials do not have the incentives to work on unrewarding tasks and tasks which are difficult to be measured. New (informal) institutions initiated from recent reforms may also crowd out the original (formal) institutions (e.g. the people's mediation 'renmin tiaojie' as an informal medical malpractice dispute resolution).

The other explanation is from the micro level. Some institutional reforms may not be as effective as expected since people's behaviour remains unchanged after these institutional reforms. If the policy implementation process is interpreted as a game, these institutional changes are not credible for players whose actions remain the same after the implementation of the institutional reforms. This explanation is consistent with the recent research in law and economics, which highlights the importance of the belief and value system.[36]

The institutional constraints of regulatory reforms as described in this book are compatible with both of these explanations. Further research is needed for detailed discussions in these two directions.

The policy areas covered in this book is listed in Table 1-1. Five policy areas will be discussed in the main body of the book, while Chapter 2 gives an overview of the Chinese health-care system, in

---

[36] Kaushik Basu, "The Republic of Beliefs: A new approach to 'law and economics'", *Policy Research Working Paper*, no. WPS 7259, 2015, Washington, DC, World Bank; Samuel Bowles, *The Moral Economy: Why good incentives are no substitute for good citizens*, New Haven, Yale University Press, 2016 and Roland Benabou and Jean Tirole, "Law and Norms", *NBER Working Paper*, 2011.

Table 1-1: The Structure of the Book

Policy Area	Topics	Chapters
Pharmaceutical regulations	Pharmaceutical sector	Chapter 3
Market regulations	Competition policy	Chapter 4
	Entry of the private sector	Chapter 7
Regulations for social programmes	Social health insurance regulation	Chapter 5
Regulations for dispute resolution	Medical malpractice dispute resolutions	Chapter 6
Public health regulations	Tobacco uses	Chapter 8

particular, the evolution of the system since the health reform in 2009. Chapter 3 discusses the regulations in the pharmaceutical sector including issues such as price control, new drug approval, essential drugs and distribution of drugs. Competition policy is expected be a very important policy area given the ever increasing economic size of China. Chapter 4 discusses the recent development of the competition policy such as anti-monopoly law and its implications for the health-care sector.

Regulatory policies in social health insurance are the focus of Chapter 5 and affordability of health care is the major policy target for social health insurance. Quality of health care is another important policy area for regulation and Chapter 6 discusses the development of resolution mechanisms for medical malpractice disputes in China. With the emergence of the regulatory state, the entry of the private sector in the health-care system is expected. Chapter 7 discusses this topic in detail. Chapter 8 focuses on an area in public health regulation, namely, tobacco control, to illustrate several important issues in public health regulation. Brief conclusions and some discussions about the implementation of regulatory policies in a broader context are presented in Chapter 9.

Chapter 2

Overview of the Chinese Health-care System

The 2009 Reform

China's most recent set of health reforms entered its eighth year of implementation in 2016.[1] Making Chinese health care affordable and accessible remains one of the top priorities of the Chinese central government. Total health expenditure reached RMB4.05 trillion, or about 6% of GDP in 2015,[2] while the annual growth rate of out-of-pocket expenditure between 2008 and 2015 hit 11.0%. Affordability of individual patients is still a serious concern. So is accessibility. Both accessibility and affordability of health-care services are serious challenges in the long term.

The 2009 reform was a product of much public debate among scholars since the mid-2000s. The debate was on whether the health system should be a health system with "direct government intervention"

---

[1] For a detailed introduction of the Chinese health-care system, see Qian Jiwei, "The Health Care System", in *Oxford Bibliographies in Chinese Studies*, Tim Wright (ed). New York, Oxford University Press, 2016. For a recent review of the health reform in China, see The World Bank Report, *Healthy China: Deepening health reform in China*, 2016, World Bank.

[2] National Health and Family Planning Commission, *Statistical Communiqué of Health and Family Planning in China in 2015*, <http://www.nhfpc.gov.cn/guihuaxxs/s10748/201607/da7575d64fa04670b5f375c87b6229b0.shtml> (accessed 24 July 2016).

or a market-oriented system. In April 2009, a compromised guideline on health reform was released by the State Council to establish a health system by 2020 in which both the state and the market would play a part.

According to the guideline, the target for the first phase of reform between 2009 and 2011 was to build a basic framework for the future Chinese health-care system while further reforms are left to the next phase. Five major components were highlighted for the first phase. First, social insurance schemes with universal coverage would be established to improve the affordability of health services. Second, an essential medicine system was to be set up for affordable and effective medicines. Third, networks of primary care clinics would be built to improve the accessibility of health-care services. Fourth, the provision of basic public health services would be equalised for all citizens. Fifth, pilot public hospitals reform would be conducted.

The first phase of health reform was formulated based on two major rationales. One was the lead role played by the government in financing, managing and providing health-care services. Financially, governments at all levels pledged to spend an unprecedentedly large amount (RMB 1.51 trillion[3]) in the health sector from 2009 to 2011. Institutionally, the government also has the means — from social health insurance programmes to publicly owned hospitals and clinics — to achieve the health-care reform targets.

The other is the spill-over effect on local pilot reforms, some of which are likely to be endorsed by the central government and implemented nationwide. For example, 200 cities had been selected for public hospital reform between 2009 and 2016,[4] which could take very different forms. Market competition will narrow down service providers in two cities while the other cities focus on hospital governance.

---

[3] <http://www.gov.cn/gzdt/2012-04/28/content_2125942.htm> (accessed 22 May 2016).

[4] State Council, April 2016, <http://www.gov.cn/zhengce/content/2016-04/26/content_5068131.htm> (accessed 22 May 2016).

Since 2009, improvements including both institutional changes and infrastructure upgrading in Chinese health-care system have been made. Between 2009 and 2015, government health expenditure growth was a hefty RMB5.9 trillion while various social insurance plans now cover 95% of total urban and rural population. Expenditure to finance operations of primary care clinics and build new primary care clinics has also chalked up big increases. However, there are still issues to be tackled including addressing the incentives of providers and insurers, and improving quality of services and medicines.

The reform has been highlighted in the 13th Five-Year Programme (FYP) period (2015–2020) with further increases in health expenditure and a reduction in the share of out-of-pocket expenditure. Further reforms of primary care providers, public hospitals, social insurance and public health are also in the pipeline.

The future development of health reform largely depends on whether the health reform takes full advantage of both market mechanism and direct government intervention. In this context, the formulation and implementation of regulatory policies are pivotal. It also depends on whether it could transfer experiences from local pilot reforms to the national level.

Health-care System before the 2009 Reform

Since the early 1980s, the Chinese government, especially the local governments, had shifted away from its policy objective of pursuing economic growth while downgrading health care to a low priority in government spending.[5] Health service providers, most of which are publicly owned, had difficulty funding health services. To make up for the shortfall, public hospitals were allowed to raise funds by selling some drugs at a 15% mark-up and providing a range of services which were not price regulated.

---

[5]Jane Duckett, *The Chinese State's Retreat from Health: Policy and the politics of retrenchment*, London and New York, Routledge, 2011.

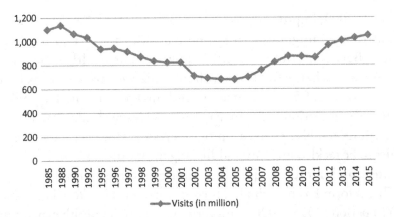

Figure 2-1: Number of Patients' Visits to Township Health Centres (in 100 million)

Source: *China Health Statistical Yearbook*, various years and National Health and Family Planning Commission, *Statistical Communiqué of Health and Family Planning in China, 2015*.

Primary care and public health service providers such as township health centres or urban community clinics, which faced difficulties in attracting patients compared to hospitals, had been underfunded to a large extent.[6] Figure 2-1 shows that patients' visits to township health centres had continued to slide from the mid-1980s to the mid-2000s.

Health insurance schemes in both urban and rural areas also did not function well. Many urban insurance schemes funded by state-owned enterprises (SOEs), which have been restructuring since 1980, were not very effective. An urban social health insurance scheme, namely, Basic Health Insurance for Urban Employees (BHI), has been initiated after the mid-1990s to replace the old insurance system funded by individual SOEs. However, as the BHI is only for urban employees who work in the formal sectors, the number of enrollees was only about 48 million in 2000, which constituted less than one third of the eligible population.[7] In the rural areas, health insurance schemes used to be supported by

---

[6] Qian Jiwei, "Building Networks of Primary Care Providers in China", *East Asian Policy*, vol. 3, no. 4, 2011, pp. 87–97.

[7] <http://www.china.com.cn/news/txt/2007-06/01/content_8328912_2.htm> (accessed 22 May 2016).

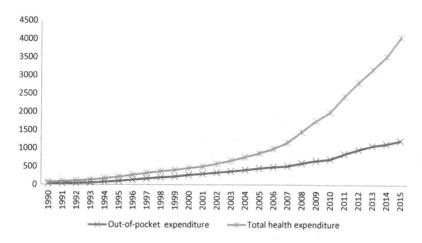

Figure 2-2:   Growth of Out-of-pocket Expenditure in China (RMB billion)
Source: *China Health Statistical Yearbook*, various years and National Health and Family Planning Commission, *Statistical Communiqué of Health and Family Planning in China, 2015*.

contributions from within a commune. However, after the 1980s, almost all rural health insurance schemes had been dissolved when household responsibility system was replaced by the commune system.

By the year 2000, the affordability issue of health-care services became so serious that out-of-pocket payment accounted for 60% of total health expenditure. Out-of-pocket payment increased from RMB26.7 billion to RMB270 billion between 1990 and 2000 (Figure 2-2). Government health expenditure only accounted for about 15% of total health expenditure. The rest of the health expenditure was funded by social insurance plans and private health insurance, among others.

Accessibility to health-care services is also a serious concern. Visits to township health centres decreased from 1.43 billion in 1981 to 0.82 billion in 2000 as many people preferred public hospitals to primary care clinics. However, supplier-induced demand in public hospitals,[8] in particular the extraordinary incentive of public hospitals to generate

---

[8]Given the nature of health services, the physician is the key decision maker during a treatment process. Supplier-induced demand refers to the situation in which the physician has the incentive to exploit profits from over-treatment or the sale of expensive drugs.

revenue by selling drugs, exacerbated the affordability issue. In 2000, revenue derived from drug sales accounted for over 46% of the revenue of a public-owned general hospital.[9]

Since 2000, some social insurance programmes have been initiated to provide financial protection for patients. For urban residents such as retirees, students, the self-employed and people working in the informal sectors, an urban resident health insurance plan was initiated in 2007, with enrollees hitting 118 million merely a year thereafter. For rural areas, a new cooperative medical scheme (NCMS) was launched in 2003, with a total of 833 million enrollees registering under the NCMS by end-2008. In 2008, over one million people were covered by insurance programmes (including the 200 million under BHI in 2008).[10]

Debates on the Direction of Health Reform between 2005 and 2009

In the early 2000s, there was a consensus among policymakers and scholars that the role of the state should be redefined and government health expenditure increased to eradicate the affordability and accessibility concerns of health-care services. After the Development and Research Centre (DRC) under the State Council released a report for formulating a Chinese health-care system in 2005, two major camps emerged.[11]

One camp which includes scholars from the DRC[12] proposes that the government play a lead role in providing and funding health-care

[9] *China Health Statistical Yearbook*, various years, Peking Union Medical College Press.

[10] *China Health Statistical Yearbook*, various years, Peking Union Medical College Press.

[11] For a detailed study of the debate between these two camps and the deliberate process of the health reform in 2009, see Yoel Kornreich, Ilan Vertinsky and Pitman Potter, "Consultation and Deliberation in China: The making of China's health-care reform", *China Journal*, no. 68, 2012, pp. 176–203.

[12] Ge Yanfeng, et al., *China Healthcare Reform*, China Development Press, Beijing, 2007.

services (a camp of "direct government intervention"). According to scholars in this camp, the main problem with the Chinese health-care system was the retreat of the state in both health financing and health provision. To them, the role of the state is pivotal to providing and financing health-care services.

Tax financing is preferred to social insurance plans given that it would be easier for the government to regulate health service provision in an integrated health-care provision system. In principle, public health and primary care services should be provided by publicly owned providers and revenue from the sale of drugs decoupled from the revenue of the public hospital. The government will have two additional tasks of equalising accessibility of health services by carefully allocating resources across regions, and defining the most cost effective treatment and medicine for service providers.

The other camp proposes the lead role of insurance programmes. This group of scholars[13] believes in universal insurance coverage for pooling risks to address both accessibility and affordability issues. Insurers, acting as a purchaser, buy services from service providers from the market. The service provider, who has to negotiate with insurers on the reimbursement rate for health-care services, will have to compete with other service providers on the basis of cost effectiveness. To address accessibility issues, private service providers will be encouraged to enter the health-care market. Market mechanisms, such as purchasing and competition, are pivotal. The role of the government is merely that of a purchaser and government health grants could be better allocated as insurance funds.

Views of scholars from these two camps have the support of different ministries. The Ministry of Health, representing the interests of public hospitals and health workers, supports views of the first camp. Together with the Ministry of Finance, the Ministry of Labour and Social Security, which is in charge of social insurance funds, supports the

---

[13] Gu Xin, "China's New Round of Healthcare Reforms", *EAI Background Brief*, no. 379, East Asian Institute, National University of Singapore, 2008.

views of the second camp.[14] An inter-ministry committee including 14 ministries was established in 2006 to set a possible direction for health reform in China.[15]

Initiatives Proposed in Guideline for Health Reform in 2009

Eight different health reform proposals by think tanks, universities and international organisations were presented to the inter-ministry committee in Beijing in May 2007.[16] The health systems proposed by these eight institutions vary between those proposed by the market-oriented and "direct government intervention" camps. After a long process of debate and revision based on these proposals, a guideline for health reform was eventually released in April 2009 by the State Council.

The target of health reform, according to the guideline, is to build a health system that will be accessible to and affordable for all Chinese citizens by 2020. As a compromise of views from the two camps, the government will play a lead role in this system while market mechanism through competition or purchasing will play a complementary role.

According to the guideline, the reform would be conducted gradually. Simpler tasks such as social insurance, establishing network of primary care clinics and local pilot reform were slated for the first phase. Tasks such as public hospital reform and payment method (between insurers and hospitals) reform, which are more complicated tasks, have to be scheduled later.

---

[14]William Hsiao, "The Political Economy of Chinese Health Reform", *Health Economics, Policy and Law*, vol. 2, 2007, pp. 241–249 and a news report in *21st Century Economic Report*, 11 April 2009, <http://www.usc.cuhk.edu.hk/Paper Collection/Details.aspx?id=7158> (accessed 22 May 2016).

[15] <http://finance.people.com.cn/GB/1037/4834237.html> (accessed 22 May 2016).

[16]These institutions include Peking University, Beijing Normal University, Fudan University, DRC, WHO, World Bank, McKinsey and Renmin University. See *Xinhua News Agency*, <http://news.xinhuanet.com/fortune/2007-11/19/content_7098474.htm> (accessed 22 May 2016).

In the guideline, the first phase of the health reform would have to accomplish five tasks between 2009 and 2011. First, achieve universal coverage of social health insurance by 2011. Second, establish an essential medicine system that will define a set of essential medicines, which are supposed to be the most effective and sold without price mark-ups in publicly owned primary care clinics. Third, set up networks of primary care clinics by upgrading the infrastructures of 2,000 county hospitals, over 30,000 township health centres and over 14,000 urban community health centres. The training of general practitioners for these primary care clinics also topped the agenda of the Chinese government.

Fourth, increase government inputs for public health services, in particular for lower income regions, to ensure equal accessibility to basic public health services across regions. Fifth, implement pilot reform for public hospitals. The reform of governance for public hospitals is highlighted. Revenue from drug sales will be decoupled from public hospital's revenue gradually. The government will increase the amount of subsidies allocated to public hospitals.

According to the guideline, the first phase of the health reform would go by two principles: Implement the five major tasks with the government playing the lead role in reform while market mechanisms will complement direct government intervention; and for all five policy arenas, local pilot programmes are encouraged and will be pivotal for future health reform.

Progress Since 2009: National and Local

From 2009 to the present, one of the most outstanding achievements made for the health reform was the dramatic increase in government health expenditure. The share of government expenditure in total health expenditure reached 30.9% in 2015 compared to 15.5% in 2000. Government budgetary subsidy per capita for public health increased from RMB15 in 2009 to RMB45 in 2016,[17] while out-of-pocket health expenditure decreased from about 40% in 2008 to 30% in 2015 (Figure 2-3).

---

[17] The State Council, <http://www.chinanews.com/gn/2016/04-26/7849120.shtml> (accessed 22 May 2016).

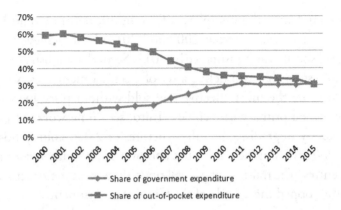

Figure 2-3: Share of Government Expenditure/Out-of-pocket Expenditure in Total Health Expenditure

Source: *China Health Statistical Yearbook*, various years and National Health and Family Planning Commission, *Statistical Communiqué of Health and Family Planning in China, 2015*.

By the end of 2011, 95% of the 1.27 billion Chinese citizens were covered by social health insurance programmes. In 2016, the government subsidised RMB420 for each enrollee under rural NCMS and urban resident plan. In August 2012, a government guideline on the "catastrophic medical insurance programme" (*"Dabing Yibao"*) was released. The catastrophic medical insurance programme is a supplementary insurance programme to extend the coverage of insurance by increasing both the rate and the ceiling of reimbursement. By the end of 2015, the "catastrophic medical insurance programme" covered over 920 million people and compensated over 3.45 million patients.[18]

In 2011, the government declared the successful establishment of an essential medicine system, in which 307 essential medicines were procured in bulk at the provincial level under a competitive bidding system and distributed to local service providers. In theory, these medicines have been selected based on the criteria of price, quality, availability and others. These essential drugs are sold to patients without any price

---

[18] China Insurance News, 10 March 2016, <http://xw.sinoins.com/2016-03/10/content_187278.htm> (accessed 24 July 2016).

mark-ups in publicly owned primary care providers. Since 2012, the number of essential medicines has increased to 520.[19]

Locally, pilot projects on the networks of primary care clinics, public hospital reform, essential medicine system and social health insurance have also been initiated. For example, in Foshan city, Guangdong province, township health centres and county hospitals have been integrated in terms of both funding and management. Primary care providers played an important part of (vertical) integrated hospitals and accounted for about 35% of total hospital revenue in 2009.[20] Similarly, since February 2008, Xiamen city has reformed the governance structure of primary care providers. All 15 community health centres in Xiamen city were merged into three public (general) hospitals. With the integrated management of hospitals and primary care providers, the referral system is expected to be improved.[21]

For the essential medicine system, the "Anhui model" is highlighted. Since 2010, the procurement office in Anhui province has been collectively procuring all essential drugs for local health service providers to provide cheap drugs. Local health service providers sold these drugs with zero mark-up. As a result, drug expenditure was reduced by 20% in primary care clinics of Anhui in 2010.[22]

For public hospital reform, the Shanghai municipal government has established a "health conglomerate" in each district since early 2011. This health conglomerate consists of a general hospital, several smaller hospitals and many community health centres. Patients have to go to a community health centre before they can visit higher level hospitals with the referral from a community health centre. Two such pilot health conglomerates were established in January 2011 in two districts of Shanghai; this institutional arrangement has been expanded to the

---

[19] Qian Jiwei and Ake Blomqvist, *Health Policy Reform in China*.
[20] <http://medicine.people.com.cn/GB/132552/188880/189037/11640591.html> (accessed 24 July 2016).
[21] Du Lexun and Zhang Wenmin (eds), *Green Book of Health Care*, Social Sciences Academic Press (China), 2009, p. 141.
[22] *Caixin* magazine, 26 December 2011.

city and some other cities have also employed similar reforms to restructure public hospitals.[23]

From May 2012, public hospitals in Beijing and Shenzhen city have removed the 15% price mark-up for the sale of drugs.[24] To compensate for the financial losses after the removal, these public hospitals increased the fee for health services. For example, in Beijing, the lowest consultation fee increased from RMB3 to RMB42 per visit. For enrollees of social insurance, RMB40 out of this RMB42 consultation fee will be reimbursed by insurance fund. Various payment method reforms have been implemented in Beijing after May 2012.

In Zhenjiang city, the pilot reform of the payment method under social insurance plans has been used for hospitals. Payment methods for hospitals such as capitation (i.e. reimbursing by the number of enrollees) and global budget have been used by social insurance plans in Zhenjiang city since 2001. Before early 2016, over 85% and 35% of social insurance plans had implemented global budget and payment by standardised clinical paths respectively. In addition, 24% of insurance plans had implemented capitation.[25]

Since 2012, in Sanming city of Fujian province, revenue from selling medicines is no longer included in public hospitals' operating revenue. The reimbursement to doctors is also not set on the basis of the revenue from the sale of drugs but by the service volume. In 2014, revenue of selling medicines accounted for about 22% of total public

---

[23] *Economic Observer*, 4 May 2011, <http://www.eeo.com.cn/eobserve/Politics/by_region/2011/05/04/200472.shtml> and <http://www.nhfpc.gov.cn/yzygj/s10006/20 1305/4fcc8e649ded4a07b78f1982f7d21a56.shtml> (accessed 24 July 2016). Similar reforms were also implemented in Yangzhou city, Jiangsu province. See <http://news.xinhuanet.com/health/2011-04/29/c_121365385.htm> (accessed 24 July 2016).

[24] *Beijing Evening News*, 26 February 2016, <http://www.chinanews.com/gn/2016/02-26/7774701.shtml> and <http://sbs.mof.gov.cn/zhengwuxinxi/difangxinxi/201201/t20120105_621533.html> (accessed 24 July 2016).

[25] See a recent State Council document, "The Opinions about Reforming Health Insurance in Urban and Rural Areas" ("Guowuyuan guanyu zhenhe chenxiang jumin jiben yiliao baoxian de yijian"), <http://www.gov.cn/zhengce/content/2016-01/12/content_10582.htm> (accessed 13 May 2016).

hospital revenue in Sanming, compared to about 37% in Fujian on average.[26]

Central and local reforms since 2009 have shown that ideas from scholars of the "direct government intervention" camp have largely set the agenda in most policy arenas including primary care clinics, essential medicine system and the provision of public health services. Market mechanisms, such as competition and purchasing, have not functioned as expected in arenas such as social insurance as well as public hospital reform during the first phase of the health reform.

Further Reforms and Remaining Issues

Subsequent reforms will build on the success of the first phase of health reform. In the 13th FYP between 2015 and 2020, government health expenditure is set to be increased further. The share of out-of-pocket expenditure in total health expenditure is expected to be reduced. There will also be an increase in the number of medicine included in the essential medicine list. Local governments have been made responsible for financing primary care clinics. The building of an information network is also in the pipeline and a patient's medical profile will be tracked with the assistance of the information system.

More importantly, the current governance structure for public hospitals will be reformed and various forms of governance structure will be tested in different localities. Social insurers will be allowed to use different payment methods including global budget, capitation and other forms to pay public hospitals. During the 13th FYP, private service providers including foreign-owned service providers are encouraged to enter the health service market.

There is however room for improvement in the affordability of health-care service. Health expenditure still increases by double digits in recent years. Annual health expenditure has surpassed RMB4 trillion in 2015. Accessibility is still a concern given the increasing imbalance of demand of health-care services in tertiary hospitals and primary care

---

[26] South Reviews (*Nanfengchuang*), no. 7, 25 March 2015, pp. 46–49.

clinics. The number of visits for primary hospitals (i.e. service providers with less than 100 beds) had increased during the 2008–2015 period by about 50 million while visits to tertiary hospitals had increased by about 876 million during same period.[27]

Outstanding issues relating to both affordability and accessibility remain to be addressed. First, from international experiences, social insurance can play an important role in controlling health expenditure, especially when the local social insurer is the major buyer of health services. However, the role of social insurer to control the growth of health expenditure is limited as reflected by the annual increase of 10.9% in out-of-pocket expenditure between 2007 and 2015 (Figure 2-2). Although some localities have pilot reforms of payment methods, many local social insurers' objective is merely to balance the budget and not to explore potential payment method reforms to control health service costs.[28]

Second, under current essential medicine system, there are some concerns regarding essential drugs selection as well as the sustainability of essential medicine system itself.[29] Patients may be reluctant to visit a primary care clinic if some medicines not in the essential list are not available in the clinic. For example, after the Anhui model was implemented in 2010, the number of visits to local township health centres has been significantly decreased. Both inpatient and outpatient visits in a township health centre in Wuhu, a major city in Anhui, decreased by 60% in 2010.[30] Under the Anhui model, primary care clinics can only sell essential medicines acquired by provincial level procurement office at the lowest price.

According to a recent nationwide survey of over 1,000 village clinics by the Chinese Academy of Social Sciences,[31] village doctors' income

---

[27] *China Health Statistical Yearbook*, various years. See also the definition of primary hospitals from Winnie Yip, et al., "Realignment of Incentives for Health-care Providers in China", *The Lancet*, vol. 375, 2010, pp. 1120–1130.

[28] See Chapter 5 of this book for a detailed discussion.

[29] See Chapter 3 of this book for a detailed discussion.

[30] *Economic Observer*, December 2011, <http://www.eeo.com.cn/2011/1227/218813. shtml> (accessed 22 May 2016).

[31] <http://www.nbd.com.cn/articles/2012-04-01/644886.html> (accessed 28 May 2012).

has decreased by an average of 50% after the restriction on the sale of essential medicines in clinics has been implemented.

Third, for recent established networks of primary care clinics, the quality of service and incentives of physicians is an important issue. Now, many primary care clinics are covered by the government budget and doctors earn a fixed salary, regardless of their service quality and quantity.[32] Doctors of primary care clinics not only do not need to maintain certain professional standard during treatment, they also tend to over-refer patients to other hospitals. The lower service quality may cause patients to visit a tertiary hospital even for minor illnesses.[33] Further, a recent study shows that the current scheme which allocates government health grant does not encourage primary care service providers to provide basic health-care services to less developed regions.[34]

Fourth, the incentive structure for public hospital physicians has not changed and health expenditure of public hospitals is on the rise. For instance, a recent study has shown that over 60% of patients in the sample are prescribed antibiotics that are not compatible with their symptoms. Even for informed patients who understand that antibiotics are not appropriate, 39% have still been prescribed with antibiotics.[35]

Figure 2-4 shows that the share of drug revenue in public hospitals remained above 35% between 2008 and 2015. Two reasons accounted for this phenomenon. On the one hand, supplier-induced demand is still expected in many hospitals given the limited role of social insurers

---

[32] For example, the visits to primary care clinics decreased in Anhui province in 2010, <http://www.nbd.com.cn/articles/2012-04-01/644886.html> (accessed 28 May 2012).

[33] Li Hua and Yu Wei, "Enhancing Community System in China's Recent Health Reform: An effort to improve equity in essential health care", *Health Policy,* vol. 99, 2011, pp. 167–73.

[34] Qian Jiwei and Young Do, "Regional Inequality in Healthcare and Government Health Grant in China", Working paper, 2012.

[35] Janet Currie, et al., "Patient Knowledge and Antibiotic Abuse: Evidence from an audit study in China", *Journal of Health Economics,* 2011, pp. 933–949.

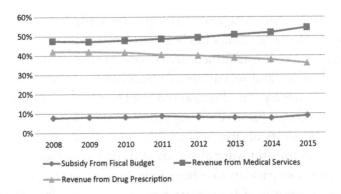

Figure 2-4: **Average Share of Different Sources of Revenue in Public Hospitals**
Source: *China Health Statistical Yearbook*, various years.

in containing the growth of health expenditure. On the other hand, reforming hospital governance structure is still a work in progress.[36]

Furthermore, since health care is a "resource dependent" and "non-productive" sector, health reform, compared to reforms in other policy areas, is even more likely to depend on the coordination amongst various government departments.[37] For example, there were 16 ministries sitting in the coordination group at the central level for health reform, which was renamed as the small leading group for health reform in 2008.[38] There are at least 11 ministries with diversified interests[39] outside of the health system which are involved in the health reform in China (i.e. Table 2-1).

---

[36] Qian Jiwei. "Reforming Public Hospitals in China", *East Asian Policy*, vol. 3, no. 1, 2011, pp. 75–82.

[37] Huang Yanzhong. *Governing Health in Contemporary China*, Abingdon and New York, Routledge, 2013, p. 136.

[38] <http://www.chinanews.com/jk/kong/news/2008/10-31/1432502.shtml> and <http://news.xinhuanet.com/fortune/2008-11/14/content_10355517.htm> (accessed 14 November 2014). From a government guideline for the tasks to be achieved for the health reform in 2013, there were 13 ministries involved in 2013.

[39] William Hsiao, "The Political Economy of Chinese Health Reform", *Health Economics, Policy and Law*, vol. 2, no. 3, 2007, pp. 241–249.

Table 2-1: Ministries Involved in the Health Reform Since 2009

Health Sector	Non-health Sectors
National Health and Family Planning Commission (including State Administration of Traditional Chinese Medicine)	Ministry of Human Resources and Social Security
China Food and Drug Administration	National Development and Reform Commission
	Ministry of Finance
	Ministry of Civil Affairs
	China Insurance Regulatory Commission
	State Commission for Public Sector Reform
	Ministry of Industry and Information Technology
	Ministry of Education
	State-owned Assets Supervision and Administration Commission
	Ministry of Commerce
	Ministry of Science and Technology

Source: Adopted from Table 1 of Qian Jiwei, "Reallocating Authority in the Chinese Health System: An institutional perspective", *Journal of Asian Public Policy*, vol. 8, no. 1, 2015, pp. 19–35.

These outstanding issues have two important implications for the future direction of health reform. First, a better understanding of the division of labour between direct government intervention and market mechanism is pivotal for the future health system. The implementation of health reform is currently included in the evaluation criteria of the performance of local officials,[40] giving local officials strong incentives to work on it. Direct government intervention is more effective for more measurable results such as infrastructure building (e.g. the number of beds) as well as providing a regulatory framework, which is the major focuses for the rest of the book.

---

[40] Karen Eggleston, "Health Care for 1.3 Billion: An overview of China's health system", *Asia Health Policy Programme working paper*, Stanford University, 2012.

The not so easily discernible and measurable aspects would be best dealt with by market mechanisms including purchasing and competition. For example, the purchase of services by insurers as a collective group of enrollees and the competition between service providers can induce hospitals to provide the most cost effective treatment and to improve on the quality of health-care services. Policymakers would do well to find an optimal mix between direct government intervention and market mechanism.

Second, there are many local pilot projects which have been conducted to deal with the aforementioned issues. However, the next big challenge is how to amass local experiences to form a nationwide model for the health system. Great efforts including careful data mining and programme evaluation of local pilot reforms are needed to identify the cause of successful or unsuccessful local pilot reforms.

Chapter 3

Regulating the Pharmaceutical Sector

Importance of Regulations in the Pharmaceutical Sector

As discussed in the introduction chapter, regulations are meant to be useful for addressing market failures where doctors have better information and knowledge of the quality and price of products than insurers and patients. In this context, there are two major reasons why a regulatory system is relevant for the Chinese health-care system. First, it is widely believed that the rapidly increasing health expenditure is a result of supply-side incentives, which refers to the situation where hospital doctors have the incentive to take advantage of their knowledge to induce more expenses from the patients and the insurers.[1] Quality of health-care services is also often overlooked. Regulations can thus improve on both the affordability and quality of the services rendered.

Second, quality of pharmaceutical products is not known to the patients and regulation on pharmaceutical products can address market failure in the pharmaceutical market. In this chapter, regulations on the pharmaceutical sector are reviewed and the degree they can address the aforementioned two points is also discussed in detail.

---

[1] For example, see a paper in a leading medical journal by Winnie Yip and William Hsiao, "Harnessing the Privatization of China's Fragmented Health-care Delivery", *Lancet*, vol. 384, 2014, pp. 805–818.

High spending on medicines and increasing health expenditure in China

As discussed in Chapter 2, affordability of health care is a very important issue. Total health expenditure in China had reached over RMB4 trillion, which accounted for about 6% of GDP in 2015,[2] compared to about 4% in 1997. Out-of-pocket payment as a percentage of total health expenditure in 2015 was about 30%. Unlike other countries, the spending on medicines is the most important component of total health expenditure in China.[3] In 2011, drug expenditure as a share of total health expenditure was 43% compared with the Organisation for Economic Co-operation and Development (OECD) average of 17%.[4] Between 2009 and 2015, the distribution market for medicines increased by more than 20% annual on average and reached over RMB1.6 trillion in 2015.[5]

The high share of expenses on medicines in total health expenditure could be attributed to health service providers' incentive to overprescribe drugs and the inefficiency of drug distribution and dispensing. After the government reduces the budget allocated to public hospitals, public hospitals were allowed to raise funds by selling some drugs at a 15% mark-up. To increase revenue, hospitals have the incentive to sell more expensive drugs for the high mark-ups.

Another reason for high drug expenditure is the inefficiency of the distribution and dispensing of pharmaceuticals. Recently, it was

---

[2]National Health and Family Planning Commission, *Statistical Communiqué of Health and Family Planning in China, 2015*, <http://www.nhfpc.gov.cn/guihuaxxs/s10748/201607/da7575d64fa04670b5f375c87b6229b0.shtml> (accessed 24 July 2016).

[3]Sarah Barber, et al., "The Reform of the Essential Medicines System in China: A comprehensive approach to universal coverage", *Journal of Global Health*, vol. 3, no. 1, 2013, pp. 1–9.

[4]Winnie Yip and William Hsiao, "Harnessing the Privatization of China's Fragmented Health-care Delivery" and OECD health statistics.

[5]<http://sczxs.mofcom.gov.cn/article/dyplwz/bh/201606/20160601332172.shtml> (accessed 9 August 2016).

estimated that on average, the retail price of a drug in a hospital in China is five times that of the producer price while the ratio is about 1.2 to 1.5 in developed countries.[6]

The Chinese pharmaceutical market is also very fragmented with over 7,000 producers and 16,000 wholesalers. In such a fragmented market, many distributors and producers give kickbacks to hospital doctors. Some local governments also pass regulations to protect local wholesalers and producers.

Regulating the quality of pharmaceutical products

Besides the extraordinary high share of spending on medicines in total health expenditure, the quality of pharmaceutical products is another concern in the pharmaceutical sector.[7] Pharmaceutical producers have strong incentives to register their products as new drugs as the price could be set much higher. It has been reported that in the year 2005 alone, China's State Food and Drug Administration (SFDA) approved the marketing of 1,113 new drugs, almost 10 times as many as the number that was approved by the US Food and Drug Administration, its American counterpart.[8] Even though some of these were generic drugs that were considered "new" because they were supplied in different dosages or packaging, those prescribing drugs in hospitals and clinics quickly began to prescribe them for the higher prices they could fetch as new drugs. In some cases, the ineffectiveness of the price regulation mechanism could be a result of corruption. Over the years, a number of SFDA officials have been prosecuted for corruption involving pharmaceutical producers; in

---

[6] National Development and Reform Commission, Economic Research Institute, "Policies and Suggestions for Reforming Pharmaceutical Distribution in China", *Review of Economic Research*, vol. 31, pp. 51–71.

[7] Elias Mossialos, Ge Yanfeng, Hu Jia, et al., *Pharmaceutical Policy in China: Challenges and opportunities for reform.*

[8] <http://news.xinhuanet.com/comments/2007-07/13/content_6364654.htm> (accessed 24 May 2016).

2007 one such case even led to the execution of a former SFDA commissioner.[9]

To address these issues, several regulatory agencies for the pharmaceutical sector have been established. The first is the NDRC, which regulates the prices for pharmaceutical products. Second, a new major regulator in this sector is the China Food and Drug Administration (CFDA), which is responsible for quality assurance for drugs and medical equipment. CFDA had been promoted from a vice-ministerial SFDA to a ministerial level agency in 2013.[10] Centre for Drug Evaluation (CDE), which is a department in CFDA, is responsible for the new drug approval.[11]

The government has employed several regulatory instruments in the pharmaceutical sector. First, local agencies of CFDA, which are independent from the local governments, have been established in all provinces, in over 70% of cities and 30% of counties. It is also expected that the approval of new drugs will be more stringent. Drugs approved earlier will be re-evaluated and the regulatory standard highlighted. In March 2016, CFDA announced that all generic drugs which were approved before October 2007 must pass clinical evaluations of their consistency by 2021.

Second, administrative interventions such as price regulation are used to control the drug price. Third, National Essential Medicine System (NEMS) has been promoted since the 2009 health reform to use cost effective medicines in primary care clinics. Fourth, reforming the distribution and dispensing system of medicine such as overhauling the procurement and bidding processes is another policy intervention. Bargaining and negotiation between social insurers and hospitals is also considered an alternative way to control drug prices.

---

[9] Yang Dali, "Regulatory Learning and its Discontents in China: Promise and tragedy at the State Food and Drug Administration", in John Gillespie and Randall Peerenboom (eds), *Regulation in Asia: Pushing back on globalization*, London, Routledge, 2009.

[10] <http://www.fda.gov/NewsEvents/Testimony/ucm391480.htm> (accessed 6 May 2016).

[11] See the document about CFDA's responsibility in the CFDA's website at <http://www.sda.gov.cn/WS01/CL0050/80623.html> (accessed 5 May 2016).

Since 2009, the essential medicine system and collective procurement system have been implemented, nationally and locally. Drug expenses as a share of total health expenditure have been reduced in primary care clinics. However, the expenses of medicine are still high and the procurement costs for medicines are still increasing rapidly in public hospitals for various reasons.

NEMS has resulted in some unintended consequences such as an undersupply of low price medicines and the underutilisation of primary care clinics. Incentives of doctors to overprescribe medicines are not addressed sufficiently. Corruption and rent seeking behaviours may emerge in the process of procurement and price setting for medicines.

Three reforms have been initiated which suggest that the government may make better use of policy interventions that are more compatible with the market mechanism. First, the government has deregulated the price control of over 2,700 medicines since June 2015. Second, the institutions for the distribution and dispensing of pharmaceuticals will be reformed. To integrate the pharmaceutical market nationwide, some regulations protecting local businesses will be abolished.

Third, further reforms in public hospitals will be initiated taking into account the structure of the pharmaceutical market. In particular, public hospitals' collective bidding and procurement platform of medicines will be implemented.

However, there are constraints as a result of limited progress in pilot public hospital reform and the lack of regulation over online drug selling platforms. These constraints are related to low capacity, regulatory agencies' lack of incentive in the pharmaceutical sector as well as some institutional arrangements in regulation.

Institutional Reasons for High Spending on Medicines

Out-of-pocket health expenditure amounted to over RMB1.2 trillion in 2015, while the annual growth rate of out-of-pocket expenditure between 2008 and 2015 reached 11.0%. Particularly for rural residents, personal health spending accounted for 9.2% of total consumption expenditure per capita in 2015 compared to 7.2% in 2009.[12]

Medicine expense is the most important component of the rapidly rising health expenditure in China. Drug expenditure accounts for about 40% of total health expenditure.[13] It is usually high compared to other countries. For example, in 2011, drug expenditure as a share of total health expenditure was 43%, higher than that of countries with similar development level (e.g. 18% in Russia and 12% in Brazil).[14] In public hospitals, drug expenditure amounted to about RMB716 billion in 2015, or 37% of the total revenue of these hospitals.[15]

There are two main reasons for the high drug expenditure. First, providers' incentive to overprescribe drugs is strong.[16] Since the early 1980s, the Chinese government, especially the local governments, has shifted away from its policy objective of pursuing economic growth while downgrading health care to a low priority in government spending.[17] After the dismantling of the central planning system, the government gradually retreated from the health sector and reduced the fiscal subsidy for these hospitals from over 60% in the 1980s to about 10% in the 2000s.[18]

---

[12] *China Health and Family Planning Statistical Yearbook 2016.*

[13] Qian Jiwei and Åke Blomqvist, *Health Policy Reform in China.*

[14] Winnie Yip and William Hsiao, "Harnessing the Privatization of China's Fragmented Health-care Delivery" and Elias Mossialos, Ge Yanfeng, Hu Jia, et al., *Pharmaceutical Policy in China: Challenges and opportunities for reform.*

[15] Calculated from Table 4-4-1 of the *China Health and Family Planning Statistical Yearbook 2016.*

[16] Janet Currie, et al., "Patient Knowledge and Antibiotic Abuse: Evidence from an audit study in China", *Journal of Health Economics*, 2011, pp. 933-949; Janet Currie, Wanchuan Lin and Juanjuan Meng, "Addressing Antibiotic Abuse in China: An experimental audit study", *Journal of Development Economics*, vol. 110, 2014, pp. 39–51.

[17] Jane Duckett, *The Chinese State's Retreat from Health: Policy and the politics of retrenchment*, London and New York, Routledge, 2011.

[18] Sun Qiang, et al., "Pharmaceutical Policy in China", *Health Affairs*, 2008, pp. 1042–1050.

As discussed in chapter 2, public hospitals and clinics had difficulty funding health services. To finance service provision, public hospitals were allowed to sell some drugs at a 15% price mark-up and provide a range of services which were not price regulated.

Primary care and public health service providers such as township health centres or urban community clinics, which faced difficulties attracting patients compared to hospitals, had been underfunded to a large extent.[19] They relied on drug revenue to finance their daily operation. In 2009, revenue from selling medicines accounted for over 50% and 44% for urban and rural primary care clinics, respectively.

Similarly, hospitals have the incentive to sell more expensive drugs for the high price mark-ups. Competition on either the price or quality does not work in the pharmaceutical sector. A recent study in China estimates that 55%-65% of antibiotic usage is driven by supply-side incentive to overprescribe and physicians have the tendency to prescribe the more expensive antibiotics.[20]

Second, another reason for high drug expenditure is in the inefficiency of the distribution and dispensing of pharmaceuticals. There were about 7,940 pharmaceutical producers[21] and more than 13,500 pharmaceutical wholesalers by 2015.[22] Each producer and wholesaler can act as a distributor of pharmaceutical products, making the market fragmented. Total market share for the three biggest wholesalers was about 33.5% of market share in 2015.[23] This share is much smaller compared to those of some developed countries. For example, the top three wholesalers accounted for 96% and 83% of pharmaceutical distribution market in the United States and the

[19] Qian Jiwei, "Building Networks of Primary Care Providers in China".

[20] Janet Currie, et al., "Patient Knowledge and Antibiotic Abuse: Evidence from an audit study in China".

[21] CEIC.

[22] Ministry of Commerce.

[23] <http://sczxs.mofcom.gov.cn/article/dyplwz/bh/201606/20160601332172.shtml> (accessed 9 August 2016).

United Kingdom in 2011, respectively. In Japan, the share was about 67%.[24]

In developed countries, value added of the distribution and retail processes accounts for about 20% to 30% of drug prices. However, in China, the same accounts for about 80% of the prices of drugs sold in hospitals.[25] For medicines sold in the retail drugstore, value added of the distribution and retail process accounts for 32% of the price of the drugs sold.[26]

In this context, drug producers or distributors of lower quality or expensive drugs may not be driven out of the market since they are competing on not only the dimension of quality but also the rents they can offer to hospitals, their major customers.

Local protectionism is also prevalent in the pharmaceutical market. To protect local businesses in this fragmented market and increase tax revenue, some local governments request local hospitals to accept bids only from local wholesalers.[27] Some local governments also impose restrictions on licence applications and insurance reimbursement for pharmacies from other provinces, making it difficult for them to open branches in their province.[28]

The dominance of hospitals is also a dampener on market competition. Figure 3-1 shows that urban hospitals and county level public hospitals accounted for over 70% of total pharmaceutical markets in 2014.[29] The large number of producers and wholesalers in the market gives hospitals even greater bargaining power.

---

[24] NDRC, Economic Research Institute, *Policies and Suggestions for Reforming Pharmaceutical Distribution in China*.

[25] NDRC, Economic Research Institute, *Policies and Suggestions for Reforming Pharmaceutical Distribution in China*.

[26] NDRC, Economic Research Institute, *Policies and Suggestions for Reforming Pharmaceutical Distribution in China*.

[27] See an example of local protectionism in the enforcement of advertising regulation for pharmaceutical industry by Markus Eberhardt, Wang Zheng and Yu Zhihong, "From One to Many Central Plans". NDRC, Economic Research Institute, *Policies and Suggestions for Reforming Pharmaceutical Distribution in China*.

[28] NDRC, Economic Research Institute, *Policies and Suggestions for Reforming Pharmaceutical Distribution in China*.

[29] <http://www.yiyaojie.com/sc/scdt/20140826/48409.html> (accessed 22 May 2016).

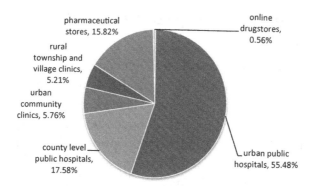

Figure 3-1: Composition of the Pharmaceutical Market in 2014

Source: Sinohealth CMH, *Blue Book for the China Pharmaceutical Sector*, 2015.[30]

To promote products to hospitals, producers and distributors usually hire sales representatives who normally provide kickbacks of about 20% of the value of the prescription[31] to hospital managers and physicians for procuring and prescribing their products.[32]

In some cases, price mark-ups for all distributors and producers, and kickbacks for hospitals amounted to as high as 10 times the producer price.[33] Producers or wholesalers could be charged for bribery or such rent-seeking behaviours. A well-known case was that of the British pharmaceutical company GlaxoSmithKline which was fined US$500 million for bribing hospitals and doctors in September 2014.[34]

---

[30] <http://www.pharm-sh.com.cn/art/2015/8/25/art_21_5363.html> (accessed 22 May 2016).

[31] Winnie Yip and William Hsiao, "Chinese Health System at a Crossroads", *Health Affairs*, vol. 27, no. 2, 2008, pp. 460–468.

[32] Tang Shenglan, et al., "Pharmaceutical Policy in China: Issues and Problems", *WHO China Pharmaceutical Policy*, 2007.

[33] NDRC, Economic Research Institute, *Policies and Suggestions for Reforming Pharmaceutical Distribution in China*; Zhu Hengpeng, "Abuses in the Health Care System and Distortions in Pharmaceutical Pricing", *Social Sciences in China*, Issue 4, 2007, pp. 89–103.

[34] *New York Times*, 19 September 2014, <http://www.nytimes.com/2014/09/20/business/international/gsk-china-fines.html?_r=0> (accessed 24 May 2016).

Three Sets of Regulatory Policies to Address High Drug Costs

Ways to curb rising drug costs will have to take into consideration the fragmented structure of the pharmaceutical market and providers' incentive to overprescribe medicines. There are three sets of regulatory policies: First is the use of the traditional method of administrative intervention such as price ceiling to reduce price mark-ups. The NDRC has set price ceiling for about 2,700 items out of about 11,000 medicines in the market for procurement and dispensing.[35]

Second is the use of the NEMS to reduce the expenses of medicines since the 2009 health reform. According to the World Health Organisation, essential medicine is defined as "those that satisfy the priority health-care needs of a population".[36] Accordingly, essential medicines are "intended to be available in functioning health systems at all times, in adequate amounts, in appropriate dosage forms, at assured quality and adequate information, and a price the individual and the community can afford".[37]

During the round of health reform which began in 2009, a guideline for establishing essential medicine system was released in August 2009.[38] In this guideline, essential medicines are defined as cost effective drugs that should be accessible to patients and serve basic medical needs.[39] The NEMS refers to a system which manages essential

---

[35] Sarah Barber, et al., "The Reform of the Essential Medicines System in China: A comprehensive approach to universal coverage", *Journal of Global Health*, vol. 3, no. 1, 2013, pp. 1–9.

[36] <http://www.who.int/trade/glossary/story025/en/index.html> (accessed 24 May 2016).

[37] <http://www.who.int/trade/glossary/story025/en/index.html> (accessed 24 May 2016).

[38] See also Ministry of Health, et al., Guideline for Implementing National Essential Drug System, 2009, <http://news.xinhuanet.com/politics/2009-08/18/content_11903865.htm> (accessed 25 May 2016).

[39] <http://news.xinhuanet.com/politics/2009-08/18/content_11903865.htm> (accessed 25 May 2016).

Table 3-1: Comparison of Different Essential Medicine Lists in China

Name	Number of Drugs	Year
National essential medicine list	2,033	2004
National essential medicine list for health insurance and work related insurance	1,850	2004
Provincial level rural social health insurances' essential medicine lists	N/A	2009
National essential medicine list	307	2009
National essential medicine list	520	2012

Source: Compiled by the author.

medicines including selection, production, distribution, dosage, pricing, regulating as well as reimbursement.

The first essential medicine list including 307 drugs for primary care clinics was released in 2009 and in 2012 the list was expanded to 520 (Table 3-1). A new version is expected to be released in 2015. However, the list had not been updated by the end of 2016. Each province also has the discretion to add or remove drugs from this list according to local conditions. On average 236 medicines were added to the provincial version of essential medicine lists, with the richer provinces adding more.[40]

All primary care clinics are required to procure essential medicines and be given priority in the prescription of primary care providers. Other service providers are also required to give the same priority to essential medicines and to meet a minimum quota in the prescription of essential medicines.

The NDRC has also set a guideline for the pricing of all essential medicines, with the provincial level government setting the local retail price. All essential medicines are to be sold without any price mark-ups in a primary care clinic.

---

[40] Sarah Barber, et al., "The Reform of the Essential Medicines System in China".

All essential medicines are covered by social health insurance plans such as Basic Medical Insurance plan for urban employees and New Rural Cooperative Medical Scheme for rural residents. The reimbursement rate is also set significantly higher than the reimbursement rate for other drugs.

According to the guideline released in August 2009, all publicly owned primary care clinics have to be equipped with essential medicines. Doctors or physicians in hospitals should also give essential medicines priority in their prescription. The target was to have at least 30% of publicly owned primary care clinics equipped with essential medicines by end 2009 and the framework of National Essential Medicines System established by 2011; by 2020, the NEMS will be fully implemented.

Third is to reform the distribution and dispense system of medicines. In particular, the building of a more centralised distribution system and a collective procurement and distribution system for both essential medicines and non-essential medicines at the provincial level are highlighted (Table 3-2).

A two-envelope tendering system is promoted for procuring essential medicines. Under this system, suppliers submit two sets of documents in the bidding process. The first set is about compliance with quality and performance standards. The second set is about the bidding price. A collective bidding system has been implemented for public

Table 3-2: Collective Bidding System for Essential and Non-essential Medicines

	Essential Medicines	Non-essential Medicines
Bidders	Producers	Producers and wholesalers
How the money is paid	Paid by the government-led platform	Hospitals
Procurement	Procurement must be made when the bidding process is over	Procurement can be separated from the bidding process
Bidding method	Two envelopes	Bidders to submit warranties for the quality

Source: Adopted from the NDRC, Economic Research Institute, 2014.

hospitals. Government-led bidding platforms have been established in all regions and the majority of counties have implemented online purchasing. Both distributors and producers can be the sellers in the bidding process.

However, the bidding and procurement processes for some public hospitals are not closely linked. Sometimes, wholesalers can renegotiate with a public hospital for procurement even after the bidding (i.e. second round price negotiation, "*erci yijia*").

Achievements and Problems of Policies Controlling Drug Prices

Considerable achievements for containing increasing drug costs since 2009 have been registered. Currently, all publicly owned primary care clinics are equipped with essential medicines.[41] After implementing the NEMS, the share of expenses for medicines in total outpatient expenses per episode in urban and rural primary care clinics had been reduced from 71.5% and 62.3% in 2009 to 68.9% and 54.2% in 2015, respectively.[42] Drug revenue as a share of total revenue for primary care clinics has also decreasd since 2009 (Figure 3-2).[43]

In public hosptials, the share of drug revenue in total health expenditure has also decreased. However, the magnitude of the changes of the share of drug revenue is relatively small. The revenue for selling drugs as a share of total hospital revenue decreased from 42.1% in 2009 to 36.2% in 2015 (Figure 2-4).

However, some issues have arisen. First, there are some unintended consequences of NEMS. Since its implementation in 2009, some

---

[41] <http://www.nhfpc.gov.cn/tigs/ygjb/201505/2f9a3505457d4179b8822c7444da2f6a.shtml> (accessed 25 May 2016).

[42] *China Health Statistical Yearbook*, various years.

[43] For a more comprehensive review of the implementation of the essential medicine system in China, see Li Lili, Qian Jiwei and Wu Xun, "A Systematic Review of Empirical Studies of Essential Medicines Policy in China: Implications for evidence-based policy making (EBPM) in developing countries", Working paper, 2016.

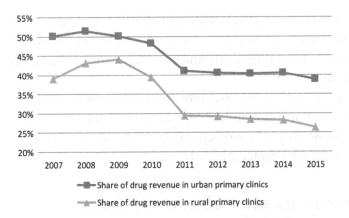

Figure 3-2: Share of Drug Revenue in Primary Care Clinics in Urban and Rural Areas

Source: *China Health Statistical Yearbook*, various years.

low-price drugs have been squeezed out of the market. At the provincial platform for collective procurement of essential medicines, the price rather than quality is the most important dimension when bidders are evaluated. Some bidding prices are so low that they cannot even cover production costs, forcing some producers of low-price medicines out of the market.[44]

Medicines included in the essential medicine list may not be able to meet the demand of patients and doctors who may prefer a larger variety of medicines. A recent research also finds that the utilisation of health-care service has decreased after implementing NEMS.[45]

Second, since the reform of public hospital is only at a very early stage, the incentives of doctors in public hospitals to overprescribe drugs remain unaddressed. Procurement costs for drugs in public hospitals have increased even after 2009. Figure 3-3 shows that in public

---

[44] <http://news.xinhuanet.com/politics/2013-06/29/c_124930012.htm> (accessed 25 May 2016).

[45] Li Kai, Sun Qiang, Zuo Gen-yong, et al., "Study of the Impact of Essential Medicine System on the Patient Visits and Cost in Township Hospital: Based on the evaluation method of difference in difference", *Chinese Health Economics*, vol. 31, 2012, pp. 62–64.

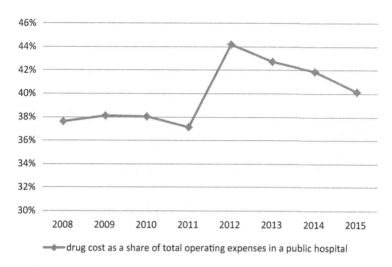

— drug cost as a share of total operating expenses in a public hospital

Figure 3-3: Drug Cost as a Share of Total Operating Expenses in a General Hospital

Source: *China Health Statistical Yearbook*, various years.

hospitals, drug expenditure as a share of operating expenses had increased from about 38% in 2008 to about 40% in 2015.[46]

Third, setting price ceiling for medicines by a government agency has resulted in rent-seeking behaviours. For example, by the end of 2014, four former high ranking officials in the NDRC who used to be in charge of setting price ceiling for medicines had been arrested for receiving bribes.[47]

Fourth, the negotiation and bargaining mechanism between social health insurers and health service providers has only been recently implemented and loopholes do exist. Social insurers are not very effective in controlling the prices of medicines, in particular patent medicines sold in hospitals.[48]

---

[46] *China Health Statistical Yearbook*, various years.

[47] <http://m.ftchinese.com/story/001059657 and http://news.xinhuanet.com/politics/2015-05/06/c_127768666.htm> (accessed 25 May 2016).

[48] *Beijing Business Today*, 14 April 2015, <http://news.xinhuanet.com/fortune/2015-05/06/c_127769545.htm> and <http://china.caixin.com/2015-03-23/100793732.html> (accessed 25 May 2016). See also the discussion in Chapter 5 on this topic.

Recent Initiatives: Deregulation and the Increasing Role of the Market

Given the issues raised earlier, since 2014, reforms of pharmaceuticals have been adjusted to implement policies that are compatible with market mechanisms. In particular, traditional price control has been deregulated.[49] Market-oriented solutions to contain drug expenditure include collective procurement of the drugs as well as bargaining and negotiation between insurers, and between purchasers and hospitals.

Since 2014, a number of initiatives have been announced and these initiatives highlight the role of the market. First, in September 2014, the Ministry of Commerce and five other ministries released a government guideline pertaining to the distribution and dispense institution of medicines. A national integrated market for pharmaceuticals is expected to be established. All regulations in conflict with Antitrust Law and Anti-unfair Competition Law (i.e. regulations to protect local businesses) should be renounced.[50]

Second, in May 2015, except for a very small number of drugs for mental diseases and anaesthetic, NDRC deregulated the price for over 2,700 medicines.[51] In the future, the prices for medicines will be largely determined by the market.

Third, a series of policies on drug procurement and sale in public hospitals have been passed. In February 2015, the State Council released a guideline on the collective procurement process for public hospitals.[52]

---

[49] See the recent policy changes to the deregulation of pharmaceuticals products, <http://politics.people.com.cn/n/2015/0505/c1001-26951137.html> (accessed 24 July 2016).

[50] <http://www.mofcom.gov.cn/article/h/redht/201409/20140900723767.shtml> (accessed 25 May 2016).

[51] <http://news.xinhuanet.com/fortune/2015-05/06/c_127768805.htm> (accessed 25 May 2016).

[52] <http://www.gov.cn/zhengce/content/2015-02/28/content_9502.htm> (accessed 25 May 2016).

The collective procurement for controlling drug costs performs two functions. It will publicise the prices to reduce the possibility of kickbacks and increase the market power of hospitals over producers and wholesalers in demand of drugs. In this case, the procurement price is expected to be lower.

In May and June 2015, two government documents were released to announce the impending removal of all price mark-ups for medicines in public hospitals in 100 pilot cities.[53] A limit of 25% to 30% for hospital spending for procuring medicines under the collective procurement system has been set.[54]

Negotiation between social insurers and health-care service providers is another mechanism to control drug prices. The reimbursement list for social insurance in 2009 included 2,151 products[55] and in principle, insurers can negotiate with providers for drug prices in this list.

To rectify the undersupply of low-price drugs, the State Council launched a series of policies to promote production of low-price drugs in April 2014.[56] These policies include nominating producers for under-supplied medicines and allowing some price mark-ups for these producers.[57]

Despite the many policies and measures, challenges remain. First, the progress of public hospital reform is still limited. The reduction of drug prices is relatively small. Although the reform is pivotal to addressing providers' incentive to overprescribe medicines by decoupling public hospitals' drug revenue from the compensation to doctors, it led

---

[53] <http://jjckb.xinhuanet.com/2015-05/18/content_547967.htm> (accessed 25 May 2016).

[54] <http://www.nhfpc.gov.cn/yaozs/s3573/201506/36a74780403d4eed96ca93b6656 20941.shtml> (accessed 25 May 2016).

[55] <http://www.mohrss.gov.cn/SYrlzyhshbzb/ldbk/shehuibaozhang/shengyu/200911/ t20091127_86904.htm> (accessed 25 May 2016).

[56] <http://www.mohrss.gov.cn/gkml/xxgk/201404/t20140422_128912.htm> (accessed 25 May 2016).

[57] <http://politics.people.com.cn/n/2014/0416/c1001-24900260.html> (accessed 25 May 2016).

to the exit of some producers and wholesalers after the revenue from selling drugs have been decreased.

For example, since 2012, in Sanming city of Fujian province, revenue from selling medicines is no longer included in public hospitals' operating revenue. The reimbursement to doctors is also not set on the basis of the drug selling revenue but by the service volume. In 2014, the revenue for selling medicines accounted for about 22% of total public hospital revenue in Sanming, compared to about 37% in Fujian on average.[58]

However, the impact of Sanming reform is still limited. For example, after the 2012 pilot reform, prices of most drugs have been decreased by 10%, significantly lower than expected.[59] In the meantime, given the relatively small market size of Sanming, which accounts for about 3% of revenue of Fujian's pharmaceutical market, some producers and wholesalers simply exit the Sanming market.[60]

Second, the limited regulatory initiatives for online transactions of pharmaceutical products posed challenges to medicinal quality. Currently, medicines from e-commerce platforms are normally more competitive in terms of pricing and save costs for consumers. Recently, the volume traded in e-commerce platforms for selling medicines has expanded very quickly.

In 2011, revenue from online drug stores was RMB400 million and in 2014, it shot to RMB7.2 billion. In 2015, the figure hit over RMB11 billion. A total of 375 firms are eligible to sell medicines online.[61]

The asymmetry between online revenue and regulation for trading medicines online is a cause for concern as the quality of medicines traded online is thus not regulated. For example, all major criminal cases selling fake drugs in Jiangsu in 2012 used the internet as the exchange

---

[58] *South Reviews* (*Nanfengchuang*), no. 7, 25 March 2015, pp. 46–49.
[59] *South Reviews* (*Nanfengchuang*), no. 7, 25 March 2015, pp. 46–49.
[60] *South Reviews* (*Nanfengchuang*), no. 7, 25 March 2015, pp. 46–49.
[61] *Caijing* magazine, 28 February 2015, <http://magazine.caijing.com.cn/20150228/3828601.shtml> (accessed 25 May 2016).

platform.[62] Although the State Food and Drug Administration solicited opinions for drafting a regulation for selling drugs online in June 2014,[63] no further development and no new version of draft were released by the end of 2016.

Constraints of the Regulatory Reform

The institutional and capacity of the regulatory agencies are major concerns in implementing regulatory policies. For example, in 2014, there were only 135 staff at the Centre for Drug Evaluation (CDE), 89 of whom were professionals working on new drug approval.[64] However, there were over 18,000 items pending approval by the end of 2014. In contrast, its counterpart in the United States has a staff strength of 3,600 staff. Under-regulation is thus prevalent in the pharmaceutical sector given the low capacity of regulatory agencies.

Local protectionism is a concern. The pharmaceutical industry is important in some localities in terms of economic development and fiscal revenue. Local regulators may favour local producers and local distributors. For example, in the procurement guideline for public hospitals in Liaoning province in 2015, it is explicitly stated that hospitals should give priority to pharmaceutical products made in Liaoning.[65]

Institutional arrangement for coordination among government departments is also a concern since a number of government departments are involved in the regulatory reform of the pharmaceutical sector. In December 2015, a regular inter-ministerial joint conference (*Lianxi Huiyi*) involving 10 ministries was held and CFDA was the coordinator of the inter-ministerial joint conference. The 10 ministries

[62] <http://www.y-lp.com/pages/Article.aspx?id=4932936417288291368> (accessed 25 May 2016).

[63] <http://www.sda.gov.cn/WS01/CL0783/100534.html> (accessed 25 May 2016).

[64] <http://stock.qq.com/a/20160425/012800.htm> (accessed 5 May 2016).

[65] <http://www.yiyaojie.com/zb/zbzc/20151105/92662.html> (accessed 30 May 2016).

involved included CFDA, NDRC, Ministry of Finance, National Health and Family Planning Commission, Ministry of Industry and Information Technology.[66] However, this regular joint conference has no enforcement power and is not expected to coordinate with the small leading group for health reform under the State Council. How to have more effective regulatory reforms involving multiple government departments is a serious issue.

---

[66] <http://epaper.21jingji.com/html/2015-12/29/content_28428.htm> (accessed 5 May 2016).

Chapter 4

Competition Policy and Enforcement in the Pharmaceutical Sector

The Competition Policy of the Pharmaceutical Sector

One very important policy area for regulating the pharmaceutical sector is the competition policy. Competition policy is an indispensable part of the regulatory framework to address market imperfection in the pharmaceutical sector for three reasons.

First is the tendency of companies to violate the rules of fair competition for gains. For example, in September 2014, British pharmaceutical company GlaxoSmithKline was fined US$500 million for bribery, a violation of Anti-unfair Competition Law (AUCL) in China.[1] Second is the inclination to abuse market power and impose constraint on competition in the area of intellectual property right, which is closely associated with the high profits enjoyed by multinational pharmaceutical companies in China. Third is the abuse of monopoly rights when setting prices of pharmaceutical products, jeopardising consumer welfare. For example, PLIVA company, a member of the Teva Group, one of the largest global pharmaceutical companies, had set the price of one

---

[1] Daniel Chow, "How China's Crackdown on Corruption Has Led to Less Transparency in the Enforcement of China's Anti-Bribery Laws", *UC Davis Law Review*, vol. 49, 2015, pp. 685–701.

of its off-patent antibiotic drugs 20 times higher than the price of its counterparts in China in 2015.[2]

Anti-monopoly law, which is the core of competition policy, is critical for correcting market imperfection and protecting consumers' interests. Currently, more than 100 countries have adopted competition law. In terms of the size of the economy and hence the volume of activities, China is now one of the major jurisdictions for competition laws in the world, behind the United States and the EU.

Since the 1980s, the government has recognised the harmful effects of monopolistic behaviour and promulgated a series of laws and regulations to address the problem. These include AUCL and price law, among others.

In 2008, the most systematic competition law, Anti-monopoly Law (AML), was enacted. Monopolistic behaviours including collusive agreement, vertical restrictions, abuse of market dominance and administrative monopoly have been defined and sanctions for corresponding behaviours specified. The AML draws from elements of both US and EU competition laws while it is more closely associated with the EU model.[3] The AML is also reflective of the political and economic conditions in China.[4]

In China, three major government agencies are entrusted with enforcing the competition policy. The NDRC is responsible for the enforcement of collusive agreements involving pricing decisions and price-related abuse of a dominant position. The State Administration for Industry and Commerce (SAIC) is the enforcer for non-price-related abuse of a dominant position and collusive agreements involving non-price coordination. The Ministry of Commerce (MOFCOM) is the enforcer for merger control provisions.

---

[2] *Yangcheng Evening News*, 12 April 2015, <http://news.ycwb.com/2015-04/21/content_20117275.htm> (accessed 25 May 2016).
[3] US-China Business Council. *Competition Policy and Enforcement in China*, 2014.
[4] Stephen Harris, et al., *Anti-monopoly Law and Practice in China*, Oxford, Oxford University Press, 2011.

Enforcement efforts have increased significantly since 2013. MOFCOM has reviewed a number of merger and acquisition cases involving transactions of major multinational companies in recent years. Since 2013, penalties under AML and the share of fines in the total turnover of involved firms have also increased significantly.

In 2013, the pharmaceutical industry was listed among six sectors as the major areas of competition policy enforcement by NDRC. Since 2015, three local health bureaus have been charged with violating AML in the process of procuring pharmaceutical products.

Competition policy enforcement has registered achievement in the reduction in consumer prices for selected products and services, such as the prices of milk powder and automobiles, and the utilisation of more economic analyses to understand the welfare impact of the monopoly practices.

Recently, a series of government regulations including new regulations for establishing national integrated market have been initiated to complement the competition policy for the next stage of economic development in China. In particular, the role of competition policy in establishing nationwide integrated market and innovation in small and medium-sized enterprises has been emphasised in these regulations. However, there are remaining important issues to be addressed including the tension between industrial policy and competition policy, the lack of capacity for the public agencies and the "regulatory capture" in which regulators represent the interests of the regulated.[5]

Monopoly as a Market Imperfection in China

Monopoly is likely to reduce consumer welfare with the increase in consumer price. In many cases, firms pursue profit by creating and strengthening a monopolistic position in the market. Monopolistic

---

[5] "Regulatory capture" was initially used by George Stigler, "The Theory of Economic Regulation", *The Bell Journal of Economics and Management Science*, 1971, pp. 3–21. For a recent review of this concept, see Ernesto Dal Bó, "Regulatory Capture: A review", *Oxford Review of Economic Policy*, vol. 22, no. 2, 2006, pp. 203–225.

firms can take advantage of their market power[6] and reduce the competiveness of the market by conducting anticompetitive actions.

These actions include collusive agreements, anticompetitive mergers and exclusionary behaviour. Monopoly conduct results in higher prices, less choice for consumers, lower output, slower innovation and economic growth.[7] In the short-term, monopolies survive due to high price not efficiency. In the long-term, monopolies have no incentive to innovate and improve.

In principle, social welfare will be reduced with these monopolistic behaviour. However, market mechanisms cannot self-regulate monopoly. Government regulation is necessary to keep the market competitive and efficient.

In China, there are two major effects of these monopoly behaviours. First, consumer price is higher with these anticompetitive actions, lowering social welfare. For example, in the telecommunication industry, it was reported that in 2011, the speed of broadband in China was only one-tenth of OECD countries on average. However, the broadband fee in China was three to four times the fees in OECD countries.[8]

Unusually high price level in the automobile industry is another example. It was reported that prices of many imported cars in China are as high as three times the retail price in the origin country.[9] Taking into account the car tariffs, the price level is still relatively high.[10] The after-sale price in the automobile industry is also high. It is estimated

---

[6]Market power refers to the case where a producer can price his/her products above marginal cost; see Jean Tirole, *The Theory of Industrial Organization*, Cambridge, MIT Press, 1988, p. 284.

[7]Massimo Motta, *Competition Policy: Theory and practice*, Cambridge, Cambridge University Press, 2004.

[8]<http://www.caijing.com.cn/2011-07-28/110791550.html> (accessed 25 May 2016).

[9]<http://finance.people.com.cn/n/2013/0821/c1004-22638569.html> (accessed 25 May 2016).

[10]<http://finance.people.com.cn/n/2013/0821/c1004-22638569.html> (accessed 25 May 2016).

that the after-sale price for a Benz car in China can be four times the average international price.[11]

Second, monopoly is associated with less innovation and slower economic growth. Recent research shows that in China when policies for improving competition in a certain sector have been targeted, the productivity of that sector is likely to be increased.[12]

One particular issue about monopoly behaviours in China which is not that common in other countries is the abuse of administrative power to create or increase market power[13] (i.e. administrative monopoly). Administrative monopoly has negative impact on consumer welfare and economic growth in China. There are three types of administrative monopoly: regional monopoly (local protectionism),[14] sector monopoly (i.e. restriction of market access to certain sector) and compulsory trading.[15]

Regional monopoly restricts market access of goods and services from the outside. In many cases, it is the local governments that create entry barriers which will segmentise the market. Local protectionism is highlighted as a major obstacle to an integrated national market in China.[16]

---

[11] <http://www.time-weekly.com/html/20140807/25956_1.html> (accessed 25 May 2016).

[12] Philippe Aghion, Cai Jing, Mathias Dewatripont, Du Luosha, Ann Harrison and Patrick Legros, "Industrial Policy and Competition", *American Economic Journal: Macroeconomics*, vol. 7, no. 4, 2015, pp. 1–32.

[13] Jean-Jacques Laffont, *Regulation and Development*, Cambridge University Press, 2015, p. 37.

[14] Xu Chenggang, The Fundamental Institutions of China's Reforms and Development, *Journal of Economic Literature*, 2011, pp. 1076–1151. Bai Chongen, et al., Local Protectionism and Regional Specialization: Evidence from China's industries, *Journal of International Economics*, vol. 63, Issue 2, 2004, pp. 397–417.

[15] Wu Changqi and Liu Zhicheng, "A Tiger without Teeth? Regulation of Administrative Monopoly under China's Anti-monopoly Law", *Review of Industrial Organization*, vol. 41, Issue 1–2, 2012, pp. 133–155.

[16] Alwyn Young, "The Razor's Edge: Distortions and icremental reform in the People's Republic of China", *Quarterly Journal of Economics*, vol. 115, Issue 4, 2000,

Sector monopoly refers to the case in which "industrial sector administrations abuse their powers by eliminating or restricting competition".[17] Compulsory trading refers to the case in which "consumers are forced to purchase goods or services that are provided by designated operators".[18]

Monopoly and the Pharmaceutical Sector in China

Monopolistic behaviours in the pharmaceutical sector in China have raised a number of concerns. First is intellectual property right. Some companies are dominant in the market because of their patents. For example, Denmark's pharmaceutical producer Novo Nordisk, with a number of patents in the area of insulin, accounted for 63% of China's insulin market in 2010.[19] The abuse of market dominance is a concern since these dominant market players may charge very high prices for the patented drugs.

Second is the high price set by companies with high market power even for those off-patent drugs. Unlike many drugs in China which come with a ceiling price set by the NDRC, prices of off-patent drugs can be set with high discretion.[20] For example, the prices of imported drugs whose patents have expired in China can be as high

pp. 1091–1135. See also discussion in a recent study, Wang Yuhua. *Tying the Autocrat's Hands*, Cambridge University Press, 2015.

[17] Wu Changqi and Liu Zhicheng, "A Tiger without Teeth? Regulation of Administrative Monopoly under China's Anti-monopoly Law"

[18] Wu Changqi and Liu Zhicheng, "A Tiger without Teeth? Regulation of Administrative Monopoly under China's Anti-monopoly Law".

[19] Reuters, 28 November 2015, <http://www.reuters.com/article/us-china-pharmaceuticals-idUSKBN0TI00J20151129> (accessed 24 May 2016).

[20] *China Youth Daily*, 13 August 2012, <http://politics.people.com.cn/n/2012/0813/c1001-18726124.html> (accessed 24 May 2016).

as five to 10 times the prices of generic drugs produced and sold in India.[21]

Third is the significant market power over procurement of pharmaceutical products enjoyed by hospitals. As discussed in Chapter 3, the share of hospitals in the pharmaceutical market is very high (over 70% in 2014). As such, hospitals have strong bargaining power in their procurement of pharmaceutical products. Commercial bribery between pharmaceutical companies and hospitals to claim market shares are common in recent years. GlaxoSmithKline (GSK) is the most high profile example.[22]

Competition Policy in China

Competition policy refers to "government policy to preserve or promote competition among market players and to promote other government policies and processes that enable a competitive environment to develop".[23] Competition law is the major policy instrument in the implementation of the competition policy[24] and more than 100 countries have adopted competition law.[25]

According to Motta (2004), competition policy serves three objectives:[26] protect consumers' welfare; protect smaller firms from

---

[21] <http://finance.sina.com.cn/consume/puguangtai/20150127/023921403245.shtml> and <http://news.sohu.com/20150216/n409043047.shtml> (accessed 24 May 2016).

[22] A couple of samples about the enforcement of US Law Foreign Corrupt Practices Act (FCPA) for bribery in the Chinese health-care system can been seen on page 34 of Wang Yuhua, *Tying the Autocrat's Hands*.

[23] UNCTAD, "The Relationship between Competition and Industrial Policies in Promoting Economic Development", 2009.

[24] UNCTAD, "The Relationship between Competition and Industrial Policies in Promoting Economic Development".

[25] Alberto Heimler and Kirtikumar Mehta, "Monopolization in Developing Countries", in Roger Blair and Daniel Sokol (eds.), *The Oxford Handbook of International Antitrust Economics*, vol. 2, New York, Oxford University Press, 2014.

[26] Massimo Motta, *Competition Policy: Theory and practice*.

Table 4-1:   The Evolution of Competition Laws in China

Competition Laws	Year	Main Emphases	Institution Enacting the Law
A regulation about promoting socialism competition[27]	1980	Addressing regional and ministerial blockade	The State Council
Anti-unfair Competition Law[28]	1993	Prohibiting administrative monopoly, below cost sales, tying and bid rigging	National People's Congress
Price law[29]	1997	Prohibiting collusion for price fixing	National People's Congress

Source: compiled by the author.

abuses of the dominance of monopoly; and promote market integration. Economic analysis is important for evaluating the impacts of a monopoly conduct over consumers' welfare level.

Table 4-1 shows the evolution of the competition law in China. The first competition law which emphasised elimination of regional and ministerial blockade in China was released in 1980 by the State Council.[30] Subsequent regulations were also released by the central government in 1982, 1990 and 2001 to address local protectionism.[31] AUCL has been enacted since 1993 to prohibit administrative monopoly, below cost sales,

---

[27] See <http://finance.sina.com.cn/g/20050418/12411526820.shtml> (accessed 20 January 2016).

[28] See <http://www.gov.cn/banshi/2005-08/31/content_68766.htm> (accessed 20 January 2016).

[29] See <http://www.gov.cn/banshi/2005-09/12/content_69757.htm> (accessed 20 January 2016).

[30] The State Council, "A Regulation about Promoting Socialism Competition" (Guowuyuan Guanyu Kaizhan He Baohu Shehui Zhuyi Jingzheng de Zanxing Guiding), <http://finance.sina.com.cn/g/20050418/12411526820.shtml> (accessed 24 May 2016).

[31] Carsten Holz, "No Razor's Edge: Reexamining Alwyn Young's evidence for increasing interprovincial trade barriers in China", The Review of Economics and Statistics, vol. 91, Issue 3, 2009, pp. 599–616.

Table 4-2: Sanctions Against Monopoly Misconduct in AML

Types of Behaviours	Definition	Market Imperfection	Sanction in AML
Collusive agreement	Collusion among firms to set price, output or market segmentation	Higher price/ lower output	Penalty between 1% and 10% of firms' turnover in the preceding financial year
"Horizontal" merger	Merger between direct competitors	Market concentration	Prohibited if it is restricting competition
"Vertical" agreement/ integration	Agreement between parties at different stages of production and distribution chain	Higher price/ market concentration	Penalty between 1% and 10% of firms' turnover in the preceding financial year
Abuse of market domination	Using the dominant position to eliminate or restrict competition	Restriction on market entry/ unfair price	Penalty between 1% and 10% of firms' turnover in the preceding financial year
Administrative monopoly	Market power is created by the abuse of administrative power	Higher price/ restriction on market entry to region/sector	Prohibited

Source: compiled by the author.

tying and bid rigging. In 1997, the price law was released to prohibit "unfair price activities" including collusion for price fixing.

However, anti-monopoly is not the major focus of these laws and regulations which did not incorporate international best practices for anti-monopoly. To fully address the concern for anti-monopoly, a more systematic competition law, Anti-monopoly Law (AML), has been enacted since 2008. EU competition law and best practices from other major countries including the United States were believed to be considered during the drafting process of the AML.

Major rules in the AML are shown in Table 4-2. Chapter 2 of the AML prohibits a range of horizontal and vertical anticompetitive agreements on price fixing, output restriction, market sharing and restrictions on products or technology developments.[32] Article 14 of the AML prohibits two types of vertical agreements: fixing resale prices and setting minimum resale prices. A fine of between 1% and 10% of firms' turnover in the preceding financial year may be imposed.

The AML prohibits firms with a dominant position to utilise it to eliminate or restrict competition. Abuses of the dominant position include unfair pricing, below cost sales, refusals to deal, exclusive[33] or designated dealing, tying or imposing other unreasonable transactional terms and discriminatory dealings. A fine of between 1% and 10% of firms' turnover in the preceding financial year may be imposed.

Under the AML, the concept of "concentrations of undertakings" includes mergers, acquisitions of control of other undertakings through purchasing shares or assets and acquisitions of control of other undertakings through contract or other means (AML, Article 20).

The AML also prohibits concentration if it has or is likely to have the effect of eliminating or restricting competition, unless the parties can prove that the concentration will lead to improvements in competition that significantly outweigh its adverse effects on competition, or that the concentration is otherwise in the public's interest.

Article 8 of the AML generally prohibits the abuse of administrative powers by public authorities to eliminate or restrict competition (i.e. "administrative monopoly").

Anti-monopoly Law Enforcement in China

Anti-monopoly law in general is enforced by public enforcement and private litigation. In China, public enforcement of anti-monopoly law takes precedence over private litigation.[34]

---

[32] <http://www.gov.cn/flfg/2007-08/30/content_732591.htm> (accessed 25 May 2016).

[33] Exclusive behaviours are defined as practices that a firm might undertake to deny a rival access to a market. See Douglas Bernheim and Randall Heeb, "A Framework for the Economic Analysis of Exclusionary Conduct", in Roger Blair and Daniel Sokol, *Handbook on International Antitrust Economics*, Oxford University Press, 2015.

[34] Zhang Huyue, "Bureaucratic Politics and China's Anti-Monopoly Law", *Cornell International Law Journal*, vol. 47, 2014, p. 671.

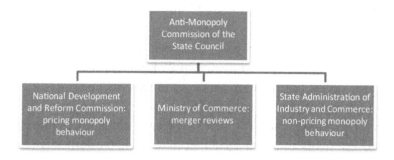

Figure 4-1:   Structure of Anti-monopoly Agencies

Source: compiled by the author.

There is a two-tier public enforcement structure for anti-monopoly under the State Council. The structure of the regulatory agency is shown in Figure 4-1. The Anti-monopoly Commission is responsible for promulgating guidelines and coordinating the work of three anti-monopoly enforcement authorities. The Anti-monopoly Commission reports directly to the State Council.

The Price Supervision and Anti-monopoly Bureau of the NDRC is responsible for enforcing the provisions on collusive agreements involving pricing decisions and price-related abuse of a dominant position, while the Anti-monopoly and Unfair Competition Enforcement Bureau of SAIC is for non-price-related abuse of a dominant position and collusive agreements involving non-price coordination. The Anti-monopoly Bureau of MOFCOM enforces the merger control provisions.

The NDRC is also charged with dealing with price-fixing and monopoly pricing while SAIC is responsible for non-price related abusive use of administrative power to eliminate or restrict competition.[35]

When the Anti-monopoly Commission of The State Council was established in 2008, the then Vice-Premier Wang Qishan was appointed as the director. Currently, Vice-Premier Wang Yang is the

---

[35] Wu Changqi and Liu Zhicheng, "A Tiger without Teeth? Regulation of Administrative Monopoly under China's Anti-Monopoly Law".

director of the Anti-monopoly Commission. Heads of NDRC, MOFCOM and SAIC serve as deputy directors.[36] Day-to-day work of the anti-monopoly commission has been assigned to MOFCOM. There is also a committee consisting of 21 legal and economics experts who provide professional advice on competition policymaking and important cases of anti-monopoly.[37]

Both the NDRC and SAIC have local branches at different levels of local governments and both agencies can delegate the authority to their local branches: local development Reform Commission and local Administration for Industry and Commerce.

All three government agencies have passed a number of regulations to complement the implementation of the AML since 2009. The enforcement of AML has significantly improved since 2013. Figure 4-2 lists the fines imposed by the NDRC on different industries since 2013. Selected enforcement cases under the NDRC are listed in Table 4-3.

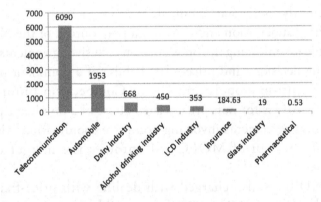

Figure 4-2: Fines Imposed by the NDRC Across Sectors After 2013 (RMB million)

Source: compiled by the author.

---

[36] <http://guoqing.china.com.cn/gbbg/2011-11/01/content_23788687.htm> (accessed 25 May 2016).

[37] <http://m.thepaper.cn/newsDetail_forward_1261301?from=timeline&isappinstalled=0> (accessed 25 May 2016).

Figure 4-2 and Table 4-3 show three important implications for the anti-monopoly enforcement. First, both domestic and foreign firms are involved in the NDRC's enforcement. Selective enforcement has been raised and foreign-owned companies are the major focus. In a survey conducted by US-China Business Council in 2014, over 56% of member companies were worried about the enforcement of anti-monopoly law. However, the cases in Table 4-3 show that both domestic and foreign-owned companies are subject to enforcement.

Second, the NDRC focuses on some sectors such as telecommunication and automobile industry for the anti-monopoly enforcement. In 2013, six sectors were highlighted as the focus of anti-monopoly law enforcement. Pharmaceutical industry was listed among these six sectors and other industries include aerospace, chemical, automobile, telecommunication and electronics.[38]

Third, both central and local enforcers are involved. For example, Jiangsu Price Bureau investigated the Mercedes-Benz case for collusive agreement in Jiangsu province.

Mergers and Acquisition (M&A) cases are reviewed by MOFCOM. The regulation for M&A review, which was released for AML implementation, stipulated two conditions. First, based on the previous fiscal year, the total global turnover for all parties to the transaction should exceed RMB10 billion and each of at least two of the parties should have a turnover exceeding RMB400 million in the PRC; second, also based on the previous fiscal year, the total turnover in the PRC for all parties to the transaction must exceed RMB2 billion and each of at least two of the parties should have a turnover exceeding RMB400 million in the PRC.

The number of cases for M&A endorsement has increased rapidly since 2008 (Table 4-4). Between 2009 and 2015, there were 1,297 cases and 1,269 cases were approved unconditionally. Only 26 cases were approved with condition. There have been only two rejected cases

---

[38] <http://news.xinhuanet.com/fortune/2013-11/24/c_118270369.htm> (accessed 25 May 2016).

Table 4-3: Selected Anti-monopoly Cases in China

Cases	Year	Country	Types of Behaviours	Sanction	Agency
Kawasaki Kisen Kaisha and six other shipping companies	2015	Japan, South Korea, Norway and Chile	Collusion and price fixing	RMB407 million; 4%–9% of annual turnover	NDRC
Qualcomm	2015	United States	Abuse of market dominance	RMB6 billion; 8% of annual turnover	NDRC
Mercedes-Benz	2015	Germany	Vertical agreement to fix prices for local retailers/ distributors	RMB350 million; 7% of annual turnover	Jiangsu Price Bureau
Dongfeng-Nissan	2015	Joint Venture (Japan)	Vertical agreement to fix prices for local retailers/ distributors	RMB123 million; 3% of annual turnover	Guangdong Development and Reform Commission
Twelve automobile parts companies	2014	Japan	Collusion for price fixing	RMB1.2 billion; 4%–8% annual turnover	NDRC
Three cement companies in Jilin	2014	China	Abuse of market dominance	RMB114 million; 1–2% annual turnover	Jilin Price Bureau
Twenty-three auto insurers and Zhejiang insurance business association	2013	China	Collusion for price fixing	RMB110 million; 0.1%–1% of annual turnover	NDRC

Six LCD[39] companies	2013	Korea and Taiwan	Collusion for price fixing	RMB353 million	NDRC
Maotai and Wuliangye	2013	China	Vertical agreement to fix prices for local retailors/distributors	RMB449 million: 1% of turnover	Guizhou Price Bureau and Sichuan Development and Reform Commission
Six dairy producers	2013	United States, France and Hong Kong	Vertical agreement to fix prices for local retailors/distributors	RMB667 million RMB: 3%–6% of turnover	NDRC

Source: compiled by the author.

[39] These firms were fined based on the Price Law rather than AML. Therefore, the amount of fine is not set on the basis of annual turnover.

Table 4-4:   M&A Reviews in China

Year	Total Reviewed	Approved Unconditionally	Approved Conditionally	Rejected
2008	20	19	1	0
2009	71	66	4	1
2010	110	109	1	0
2011	168	164	4	0
2012	164	158	6	0
2013	207	203	4	0
2014	245	240	4	1
2015	312	310	2	0
Total	1,297	1,269	26	2

Source: *China Commerce Yearbook*, various years.

by MOFCOM since 2009 (i.e. A P Møller-Maersk A/S and MSC Mediterranean Shipping Company with CMA CGM SA in 2014 and Coca-Cola company with Huiyuan Juice in 2009). The conditions imposed by MOFCOM include divestiture of assets, information firewall and mandatory licensing.

As of March 2015, there were 47 cases investigated by SAIC and 13 cases had been closed.[40] Among these cases, most are related to collusion and abuses of market dominance. Business associations were also involved in at least nine cases for collusion.[41]

A company may go for litigation against monopoly behaviours of other companies and government agencies according to the AML. The number of private litigations has increased since 2008 (Table 4-5). There were only 10 anti-monopoly cases accepted in 2008 and 2009.

---

[40] <http://finance.people.com.cn/n/2015/0309/c1004-26661326.html> (accessed 25 May 2016).
[41] <http://china.caixin.com/2013-07-30/100562532.html> (accessed 25 May 2016).

Table 4-5: Anti-monopoly: Private Litigation in China

Year/s	First-instance Cases Accepted by Courts	First-instance Cases Adjudicated by Courts
2008–9	10	6
2010	33	23
2011	18	24
2012	55	49
2013	72	69
Total	188	171

Source: US-China Business Council, *Competition Policy and Enforcement in China*, 2014.

In 2013, the number of private litigation cases increased to 72. Administrative monopoly cases can also be addressed by private litigation. Guangdong Department of Education was sued by a Shenzhen company for abuse of administrative authority for compulsory trading.

The number of cases of administrative monopoly is limited. There are only six adjudicated cases reported as at November 2015 (Table 4-6). Similar to other areas of anti-monopoly law enforcement, the pharmaceutical sector is also highlighted in the administrative monopoly area. Three of six cases occurred in the process of local health bureau's collective procurement of pharmaceutical products for local health service providers. NDRC reported that health and family planning bureaus in Sichuan province, Zhejiang province and Bangbu municipality had procured pharmaceutical products in favour of local based companies.[42] However, there is no penalty involved in administrative monopoly except prohibit.

---

[42] <http://www.sdpc.gov.cn/gzdt/201511/t20151102_757334.html> and <http://www.sdpc.gov.cn/fzgggz/jgjdyfld/fjgld/201508/t20150826_748684.html> (accessed 9 August 2016).

Table 4-6: Administrative Monopoly

Case	Year	Reason	Sanction	Enforcer
Yunnan Communication Administration	2015	Sector monopoly: collusion with local operators	Prohibit and rectify	Yunnan Development and Reform Commission
Shandong Department of Transportation	2015	Regional monopoly	Prohibit and rectify	NDRC
Guangdong Department of Education	2015	Compulsory trading	Prohibit	Guangzhou Municipal Intermediate People's Court
Sichuan and health and family planning bureau	2015	Regional monopoly	Prohibit and rectify	NDRC
Zhejiang health and family planning bureau	2015	Regional monopoly	Prohibit and rectify	NDRC
Bangbu health and family planning bureau, Anhui province	2015	Regional monopoly	Prohibit and rectify	NDRC

Source: compiled by the author.

Achievements of Recent Developments of Competition Policy in China

In terms of the size of the economy, China has now become one of the major jurisdictions for competition laws in the world, together with the United States and the EU. MOFCOM has reviewed a number of M&A cases among major multinational companies including Bev-Anheuser Busch (2009), Western Digital-Hitachi (2012), Google-Motorola (2012), Marubeni-Gavilon (2013) and Thermo Fisher-Life Technologies (2014).[43]

The enforcement effort for anti-monopoly has increased significantly in recent years. In particular, since 2013, both the amount of

---

[43] US-China Business Council, *Competition Policy and Enforcement in China.*

fine under anti-monopoly law and the share of fine in total turnover of involved firms have increased significantly. The average range of the fine as a share of turnover increased from around 1–2% in 2013 to 4–8% in 2014.

One highlighted case involves US telecommunication firm Qualcomm. In February 2015, a penalty of RMB6 billion was imposed by the NDRC on Qualcomm, about 8% of the company's 2013 China revenue, for abuses of market dominance.[44] It is the biggest fine imposed under China's AML after its enactment in 2008.

Two major achievements of the enforcement are discernible. First, consumer prices in some sectors have decreased. The fees for automobile after-sales have significantly reduced for brands Audi and Mercedes-Benz.[45] Price for over 10,000 products of Mercedes-Benz was reduced by 15% on average.[46] Milk powder brand Wyeth reduced retail price by 11% on average after NDRC's investigation.

Second, consistent with international best practices,[47] more economic analyses are used in the enforcement and implementation of anti-monopoly law. More rigorous economic analyses have been applied in the merger review. For example, comparing the two rejected M&A cases, MOFCOM applied the rule of reasons to evaluate the impact on market structure by using price increase forecast and market concentration ratios (Table 4-7).

For example, for the merger case of Coca-Cola/Huiyuan in 2009, there were no quantitative evidences shown in the final report from MOFCOM. In contrast, for the case of MSC Mediterranean Shipping Company and CMA CGM SA, MOFCOM reports market share for

---

[44] <http://finance.sina.com.cn/chanjing/gsnews/20150317/040421735797.shtml> (accessed 25 May 2016).

[45] <http://news.163.com/15/0813/13/B0TD7F9B00014AED.html> (accessed 25 May 2016).

[46] <http://www.time-weekly.com/html/20140807/25956_1.html> (accessed 25 May 2016).

[47] William Kovacic and Carl Shapiro, "Antitrust Policy: A century of economic and legal thinking", *The Journal of Economic Perspectives*, 2000, pp. 43–60.

Table 4-7: Two Rejected Cases for M&A Reviews

Case	Year	Sector	Country	Reason of rejection	Evidences
AP Moller — Maersk A/S, MSC Mediterranean Shipping Company and CMA CGM SA	2014	Shipping	Denmark and France	Significantly increased the degree of concentration and barriers to entry are significantly increased	Market share was reported; before and after merger market concentration index was reported
Coca-Cola company and Huiyuan Juice	2009	Soft drink	United States and China	Significantly increased the degree of concentration	No quantitative evidences

Source: compiled by the author.

all involved parties. MOFCOM also calculated the market concentration index (HHI) before and after merger. It concludes that the merger will change the market structure significantly and market competitiveness will be reduced.

Recently, the competition policy has been highlighted as an important policy leverage for promoting structural changes in the Chinese economy. A series of regulations have been released to complement the competition policy. First, a guideline was released by the State Council in November 2014 to address administrative monopoly in order to build up a nationwide integrated market.[48]

According to this new regulation, all firms must follow the national tax code and local governments are no longer allowed to offer tax breaks to firms without the endorsement of the State Council. Land and other state-owned assets are now not transferrable to enterprises at below market prices. Local policies that subsidise enterprises in various forms such as the waiving of utility fee are banned.

Second, in March 2015, the Central Committee of the CCP and State Council released a guideline for innovation-driven development strategy. In this guideline, the role of anti-monopoly in encouraging innovations, especially from small and medium-sized enterprises, has been specified.[49]

Third, in August 2015, the State Council released a guideline on advancing the domestic distribution of goods to make the distribution sector a new driving force for economic growth. Central and local governments are required to facilitate the formation of an integrated national market by eliminating market allocation barriers and breaking up industry monopolies.

In this guideline, the State Council requested local governments to improve antitrust enforcement and strengthen reviews for mergers. Regional trade barriers, anticompetitive agreements, abuse of market dominance and administrative power, as well as the imposition of unfair charges or conditions have to be strictly prohibited.

---

[48] <http://www.gov.cn/zhengce/content/2014-12/09/content_9295.htm> (accessed 29 August 2015).
[49] <http://news.xinhuanet.com/politics/2015-03/23/c_1114735805.htm> (accessed 25 May 2016).

Fourth, to guide the enforcement of the AML, six guidelines for enforcing anti-monopoly law are being drafted by the NDRC. These guidelines address important issues including guidelines for abuses of intellectual property right, anti-monopoly for automobile industry, leniency, amnesty, penalty calculation and breakdown process of anti-trust investigation.[50]

Enforcement against abuses of intellectual property right is particularly relevant for the pharmaceutical sector. In December 2015, a draft of the guideline to enforce AML on the abuse of intellectual property right has been published in the website of the NDRC and the public's suggestions were solicited.[51] According to a recent report, up to 2015, the pharmaceutical sector accounted for about 10% of all cases related to the abuse of intellectual property right.[52]

Fifth, a draft of the amendment of the AUCL has been published on the website of the State Council to solicit opinions and suggestions between February and March 2016.[53] Some articles which are not consistent with the AML and other laws have been amended in this draft.

Enhance Consistency and Effectiveness in Enforcing Competition Policy

While China could draw valuable lessons from developed countries on the implementation of the competition law, the implementation faces many challenges in China. First is the need to improve the capacity of these government regulatory agencies, in particular in terms of human resources. In the NDRC, there are 46 people working on the enforcement

---

[50] <http://news.xinhuanet.com/finance/2015-06/18/c_127928081.htm> (accessed 25 May 2016).
[51] <http://www.sdpc.gov.cn/gzdt/201512/t20151231_770313.html> (accessed 23 May 2016).
[52] <http://finance.sina.com.cn/china/20151103/020623656652.shtml> (accessed 23 May 2016).
[53] <http://www.chinalaw.gov.cn/article/cazjgg/201602/20160200480277.shtml> (accessed 23 May 2016).

of anti-monopoly law, while there are 40 over at the SAIC and 35 in MOFCOM for antitrust enforcement.[54] This is grossly understaffed as compared to that of the United States and the EU. For example, there were over 1,100 employees in the Federal Trade Commission, one of the two major agencies for antitrust enforcement in the United States.

Professional capacity of the enforcement is also in question. Rapid technological change and the technology-intensive nature of some industries have made it difficult for the enforcers to make a decision when reviewing M&A cases and make a judgement on the market dominance. For example, China was the last jurisdiction to approve the case about Google's acquisition of Motorola, which was cleared only on the last day of the review period.[55] While Dell's US$60 billion buyout of EMC in 2016 has been approved by the United States and EU antitrust regulators, it may still be delayed since it has not been approved by China's antitrust regulator.[56]

Second is the need to address the institutional arrangement of regulatory agents. The division of labour among government regulatory agencies and between sectorial regulator and anti-monopoly law enforcers needs to be clarified in the future. At the moment, price related cases are to be investigated by the NDRC and non-price related by the SAIC. However, some grey cases that relate to both price and non-price issues often face coordination problems between three government enforcement agencies.

Some sectors such as telecommunication and pharmaceutical industries have their own regulator. For example, the telecommunication industry is highlighted as one of the six industries for enforcing the AML. However, the Ministry of Industry and Information Technology

---

[54] Angela Zhang Huyue, "Bureaucratic Politics and China's Anti-Monopoly Law", *Cornell International Law Journal*, vol. 47, 2014, p. 671.

[55] <http://www.bloomberg.com/bw/articles/2012-03-21/why-china-is-holding-up-the-google-motorola-deal> and <http://www.theguardian.com/technology/2012/may/21/china-google-approval-motorola-mobility> (accessed 25 May 2016).

[56] <http://siliconangle.com/blog/2016/07/19/emc-shareholders-bless-60-billion-dell-buyout-next-up-chinas-regulators/> (accessed 9 August 2016).

(MIIT) is responsible for regulating telecommunication. The division of labour between the sectorial regulator and agencies for the AML thus needs to be settled. Similarly, CFDA is the government agency responsible for regulating the pharmaceutical sector.

Third is the conflict between the assigned tasks of regulators and the incentives of regulators. For example, the tension between industrial policy and competition policy should be carefully deliberated. China has employed industrial policies to promote economic growth since the 1980s. An effective industrial policy requires competitive markets; to some degree, promoting domestic firms and SOEs as one of the objectives of industrial policy in China is in conflict with the competition policy.

Since the 2000s, the Chinese government has increased its support of big SOEs (i.e. "national champions") through subsidies, protectionism and preferential procurement policies in strategic industries, including automobile and telecommunication.[57] For the pharmaceutical sector, industry consolidation has been encouraged in the 12th FYP where market share of the top 100 companies in the pharmaceutical industry had been targeted to reach 50% by 2015, compared to 40% in 2005.[58] How to justify these industry policies from the perspective of the competition policy is a tricky issue.

The tension between these two policies also reflects structural problems in the enforcement. NDRC is the major agency for both industrial policymaking and enforcing the competition policy, while the Industry Coordination Bureau under the NDRC is responsible for industrial policymaking. On the other hand, the Price Supervision and Antimonopoly Bureau under the NDRC is tasked with enforcing the antimonopoly policies. The NRDC is thus both the enforcer of industrial and competition policies.

---

[57] Thomas Hemphill and George White, "China's National Champions: The Evolution of a National Industrial Policy — or a New Era of Economic Protectionism?" *Thunderbird International Business Review,* vol. 55, no. 2, 2013, pp. 193–212.

[58] Elias Mossialos, Ge Yanfeng, Hu Jia, et al., *Pharmaceutical Policy in China, Challenges and Opportunities for Reform.*

Fourth is the conflict of interest between the regulatory agency and the violating firms. One eminent case is that of Professor Zhang Tingzhu, a member of the expert committee under the State Council assigned for the drafting of the AML. Professor Zhang was hired by Qualcomm to prove that the company did not violate the antitrust law.[59] He was eventually dismissed from the expert committee for the conflict of interest.

Fifth is with the enforcement of the AML on administrative monopoly. Currently, government agencies for enforcing the AML can only suggest the existence of violation, but rarely was the law enforced. The law could hardly be enforced as other government agencies such as local governments are themselves a participant of administrative monopoly.[60]

---

[59] <http://renwu.people.com.cn/n/2014/0912/c357678-25648568.html> (accessed 25 May 2016).
[60] *Legal Daily*, 16 February 2015.

Chapter 5

Regulating Social Health Insurance

The Development of Social Health Insurance and the Role of Regulation

In the late 1990s, over 40% of urban residents and around 80% of rural residents were not covered by any insurance scheme.[1] Since the 1990s, China has introduced social health insurance schemes that now cover more than 1.2 billion people, or 95% of the total population in China. Reimbursement from social health insurance accounted for 29.9% of total health expenditure in 2015, compared to 18.4% in 2008.[2]

Social health insurance in China comprises three major plans: Basic Health Insurance for urban employees, NCMS for rural residents and Urban Resident Basic Medical Insurance (URI) for urban residents. China's social health insurance schemes unlike that of other countries have a few peculiarities. First, all social insurance schemes in China are managed by the local government. Second, the state government and lower level governments subsidise NCMS and URI according to the number of enrollees. These subsidies are allocated in the manner of a matching grant, that is, the central government's grant must be matched with funds from the local government. Third, enrolment in NCMS and URI is voluntary.

---

[1] *China Health Statistical Yearbook*, various years.
[2] Calculated from *China Health Statistical Yearbook* and *Statistical Communiqué on Human Resources and Social Security in China*, various years.

The Chinese government has set the reform agenda between 2015 and 2020 (i.e. the 13th Five-Year Plan) for various social health insurance schemes. Coverage of social health plans will then be universal, with the government subsidising at least RMB360 per enrollee for NCMS and URI in 2015. By 2020, reimbursement rate for inpatient service would reach at least 75% and commercial insurers are encouraged to provide supplementary health insurance. Full portability of social insurances across regions would also be implemented gradually.

With the increasingly important role of social health insurance, regulations are critical for increasing financial coverage, curbing cost escalation and improving quality control. In particular, regulating the rules for reimbursement is necessary to avoid abuse by patients and hospitals and to improve the efficiency of the fund. The lack of regulation will lead to concerns for the sustainability of the social health insurance fund, which may result in conservative reimbursement rates.

Pilot projects for social insurance are being conducted in many localities. In particular, the traditional fee-for-service payment system at county level hospitals in 311 counties nationwide from late 2012 would be replaced by various alternative payment methods to control cost in hospitals. Payment method reforms have been widely implemented in China. Before early 2016, over 85% and 35% of social insurance plans had implemented global budget and payment by standardised clinical paths respectively. In the same period, 24% of insurance plans had also implemented capitation.[3]

However, social insurance has yet to implement reimbursement rules and set the financial conditions of social insurance fund. Given their incentive structure and relatively low capacity, relying on social insurers to protect patients financially and improve the quality of service still play a limited role as the financial coverage is still low for many social insurance plans.

---

[3] <http://www.gov.cn/zhengce/content/2016-01/12/content_10582.htm> (accessed 13 May 2016).

Development of Social Health Insurance: Between the Mid-1990s and Early 2000s

Before 1980, health-care funding in China provided almost everyone with access to at least one basic standard of care. In urban areas, hospitals were owned by either the state or by large SOEs. Workers and their dependents, and retirees, also had access to subsidised care through their employers (the government or a SOE). Fees charged were maintained at very low levels and funded largely by the employers or came in the form of direct state subsidies. Government Insurance Scheme (GIS) covered government employees and their dependents, while the Labour Insurance Scheme (LIS) covered SOE workers and (with reduced benefits) their dependents.

Residents in the countryside belonged to an agricultural commune and had access to basic primary care and (on referral) hospital care at low out-of-pocket charges. Under the Cooperative Medical Scheme (CMS), every commune member contributed a small amount of money as collective funds. Primary-care providers were paid by the commune, and hospitals were funded by subsidies from the central and local governments and reimbursement from the CMS.

After the dissolution of the central planning system in the 1980s, the Chinese government gradually retreated from the health sector. In urban areas, many SOEs were privatised, reorganised, or even closed. With reducing profitability, SOEs have difficulties financing health care. Financial coverage for urban residents declined significantly. In the rural areas, the commune model of organising agricultural production was replaced by the "Household Responsibility System" under which land is allocated to individual families and production and marketing decisions are decentralised to the family level. The collective fund mechanism to finance health care was no longer sustainable and CMS was gradually phased out.

A new Basic Health Insurance for Urban Employees (BHI) scheme was initiated in the mid-1990s for urban employees in formal sectors based on simple principles. First, risk-pooling and plan management is conducted through the social security bureau at the city level. Second,

Table 5-1:   Extent of Health Insurance Coverage (%)

	Urban			Rural		
	2003	1998	1993	2003	1998	1993
BHI*	30.4	N/A	N/A	1.5	N/A	N/A
GIS/LIS	8.6	38.9	66.41	0.3	1.7	3.41
CMS	6.6	2.7	1.62	9.5	6.6	9.81
Other social insurance	2.2	10.9	4.44	1.2	3.0	2.34
Private insurance	5.6	3.3	0.25	8.3	1.4	0.33
No insurance	44.8	44.1	27.28	79.0	87.3	84.11

Source: National Survey on Health Service in 1993, 1998 and 2003.

the basic version of the plan covers only current and retired employees (but not their dependents) of participating employers, be they the government, SOEs, or private firms. The intention was to gradually replace the GIS and LIS plans with the BHI and make it compulsory; this goal has so far only been partially met. By 2002, there were less than 100 million enrollees in BHI, accounting for less than 20% of total urban residents

Table 5-1 shows the insurance coverage status of residents in 1993, 1998 and 2003. Health insurance coverages in both urban and rural areas were at a very low level. Over 40% of residents in urban areas and around 80% of residents in rural areas were not covered by any insurance scheme even in 2003, almost 10 years after BHI has been introduced.[4]

Funding of the plan is through payroll deductions based on a minimum of 8% of the worker's salary (6% from the employer and 2% from the employee). This amount is then split between a "social pooling account" and an "individual account" in the name of the worker for paying both outpatient and inpatient care. This arrangement is similar

---

[4] Based on a national level survey data, the coverage of health insurance in urban and rural areas in 2000 were 38.8% and 12.6%, respectively. See Yan Yifei, Qian Jiwei and Wu Xun, "Inequalities in Health Care in China 1991–2011: Evidence from the China health and nutrition survey", Working paper, 2016.

to the Singaporean system of Medisave accounts. In the early version of the plan, the split was 3.8% to the individual account and 4.2% to the social pooling account. When an individual has an illness which requires inpatient care, he or she can seek reimbursement from the social pooling account subject to a locally determined co-insurance rate and to an upper limit equivalent to six times the average annual wage of the city.

There are however two important constraints: the deduction covers only drugs and procedures on the Essential Medicines and Essential Services list,[5] and reimbursement is only applicable for services rendered by approved hospitals and clinics under the city's social security bureau.

BHI terms however vary across provinces. Some cities with good fiscal capacity offer relatively generous benefits and complementary social insurance for BHI enrollees is also offered to improve financial coverage for patients. In Shanghai, for instance, in the mid-2000s an employer contributed 10% of income while the employer's contribution was as low as 3% in some localities in comparison with the national average of about 7.4%.[6]

By year 2000, out-of-pocket payment accounted for 60% of total health expenditure. Between 1990 and 2000, out-of-pocket expenditure increased by 900%. Government health expenditure only accounted for about 15% of the total in 2000. The rest of the health expenditure was funded by social insurance plans and private health insurance, among others.

Since 2002, NCMS has been initiated in many rural places in China under the management of the local health bureau. Unlike BHI, NCMS is a voluntary plan.[7] To attract enrolment and improve the benefits of NCMS, the central government has provided subsidies to the NCMS.

---

[5] Local government has some discretion to change items in the list.

[6] <http://www.npc.gov.cn/npc/zt/2008-12/23/content_1463573.htm> (accessed 25 May 2016).

[7] Local governments may have the incentive to encourage local residents to join social insurance plans. See Qian Jiwei and Ake Blomqvist, *Health Policy Reform in China.*

It has also specified the (minimum) individual contribution level as well as the amount of government subsidy. The allocation of subsidy is based on the condition that the local government has made sufficient contribution (i.e. matching grant). Local governments are however free to increase the government subsidy beyond the minimum level. Minimum government subsidy per enrollee (from both central and local governments) increased from RMB10 in 2003 to RMB420 in 2016.[8]

For example, in 2015, the central government set the minimum premium per enrollee at RMB500 (i.e. an individual contributes RMB120 and the various levels of government would foot the rest of the RMB380) (Figure 5-1). In Shanghai, the premium was RMB1,800, while the government is responsible for over four-fifths of the bill in 2015.[9] In terms of the premium, regional difference is huge. For 2015, most plans in Hubei province had set the premium at RMB500, the minimum level set by the state guideline.[10]

NCMS is designed and managed by county governments but subject to broad principles set by the state. In some aspects it functions in the same way as urban BHI plans. In others, what is covered under the NCMS is limited to the same services and drugs covered in BHI plans; there are also others who divide their funds into the equivalent of individual accounts and a county-wide social pooling account.

NCMS focuses on the financial protection of inpatient services. However, as the resources of the plans are limited, out-of-pocket expenditure for NCMS enrollees was as high as 50% for inpatient services in 2015.[11] The plan also has a rather low maximum pay-out per

---

[8] National Health and Family Planning Commission, <http://www.chinanews.com/gn/2016/05-06/7860162.shtml> (accessed 12 May 2016).
[9] For example, see the document released in the Jinshan district, Shanghai, <http://wsj.jinshan.gov.cn/html/hzyl/zcfg/635507383918.html> (accessed 12 May 2016).
[10] <http://www.nchzyl.cn/detail_20151110101945000001.html> (accessed 12 May 2016).
[11] *Jiankang Bao*, 18 November 2015, <http://www.jkb.com.cn/news/depth/2015/1118/380469.html> (accessed 13 May 2016).

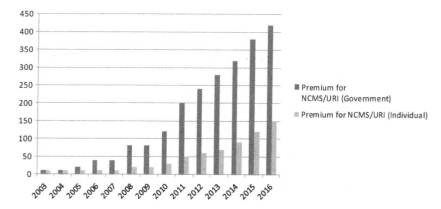

Figure 5-1: (minimum) Government Subsidy (RMB) Per Enrollee Under NCMS/URI from 2003 to 2016*

Source: China Health Statistical Yearbook and Statistical Communiqué on Health and Family Planning in China, various years.

year or per visit. NCMS thus offers considerably less complete insurance protection than the BHI plans.

By 2007, there were over 70% of urban residents who were not covered by BHI.[12] Urban Resident Health Insurance (URI) was initiated in 2007 to cover those not covered by BHI, including retirees, self-employed, students and others. URI is modelled on the NCMS — voluntary and managed by the local social security bureau which sets the local URI policy at the city level.

Like other social health insurance schemes, local variation of health policy for URI is also large. For example, in Shanghai in 2011, the premium for those aged 70 or above was RMB1,500 while government's subsidy was RMB1,260 per enrollee.[13] Reimbursement rate varies from 50% to 80% depending on the hospital's grade. In Lanzhou city, Gansu province, in 2011, the premium per enrollee was set at

---

[12] BHI covered only 53% of employees in urban areas in 2007.
[13] <http://www.zgylbx.com/pNMalvXRKUaInew17408_1/> (accessed 25 May 2016).

RMB160 while government subsidised RMB80.[14] The reimbursement rate varied from 50% to 65% and at a ceiling of RMB18,000.

While social insurance schemes in other countries are run by non-profit organisations or independent government bureaus, those in China are usually managed by the local government at the city/county level. In particular, BHI and URI are managed by the local social security bureau, while NCMS is handled by the local health bureau.[15] Both the local health bureau and social security bureau report to the local government. This implies that the benefits and policies of the social insurance schemes may differ in different places.[16]

Inpatient claims in Shanghai were applicable to expenses in excess of RMB1,500 up to a maximum of RMB390,000 in 2015. Within this range, the reimbursement rate was 80% or even higher. Anything in excess would require the BHI enrollee to buy complementary social insurance which will cover 80% of health expenditure.[17] In Xi'an, the ceiling is set at RMB400,000 under complementary social insurance for BHI enrollees in 2016 and the co-insurance rate is about 5-20% (social insurance's coverage is 80%-90%). Patients will have to foot the bill entirely at 100% for anything in excess of the ceiling.[18]

Unlike social health insurance in other countries, NCMS and URI are voluntary rather than compulsory. The premium is not based on community rating of risk but set by the local government based on available budget. For many social insurance plans, various levels of government subsidy are allocated in the manner of matching grant.

---

[14] <http://www.lanzhou.gov.cn:8080/root84/srmzfbgt/201105/t20110520_40845.html> (accessed 25 May 2016).

[15] In some cities, such as Tianjin, URI and NCMS are being integrated.

[16] See Mok Ka-Ho and Qian Jiwei, *A New Welfare Regime in the Making? Paternalistic Welfare Pragmatism in China*, 2016, for an analysis of the role of local government from a broader perspective in social policy implementation.

[17] <http://shanghai.chashebao.com/wenti/14094.html> (accessed 25 May 2016).

[18] <http://www.xahrss.gov.cn/appeal/list2.jsp?tm_id=75&model_id=2&sq_title=&cur_page=21&pur_id=4> (accessed 25 May 2016).

Achievements of the Social Health Insurance Scheme

By the end of 2011, 95% of Chinese citizens were covered by one of the social health insurance plans (see Figures 5-2 and 5-3). In 2016, the government will subsidise RMB420 for each enrollee under rural NCMS and URI plans.[19]

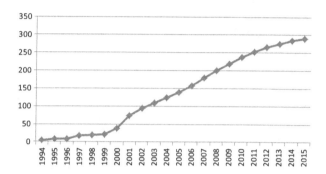

Figure 5-2: Number of Enrollees Under BHI (million)

Source: China Health Statistical Yearbook, various years and *Statistical Communiqué on Human Resource and Social Security in China 2015.*

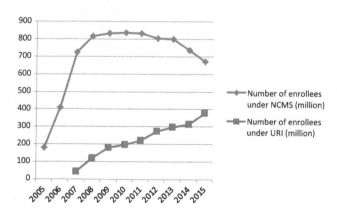

Figure 5-3: Number of Enrollees in NCMS and URI (million)

Source: China Health Statistical Yearbook, various years, *Statistical Communiqué on Human Resource and Social Security in China, 2015* and *Statistical Communiqué on Health and Family Planning in China 2015.*

---

[19]<http://www.mof.gov.cn/zhengwuxinxi/zhengcefabu/201605/t20160506_1978682.htm> (accessed 13 May 2016).

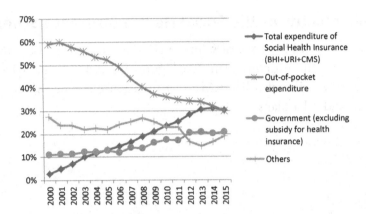

Figure 5-4: Composition of Health Expenditure in China

Source: China Health Statistical Yearbook, various years, *Statistical Communiqué on Human Resource and Social Security in China, 2015* and *Statistical Communiqué on Health and Family Planning in China, 2015.*

Figure 5-4 shows a continuously decreasing trend for out-of-pocket expenditure and an increasing government input for health care, much of which is used to subsidise social insurance claims.

In 2015, reimbursement from all social health insurance schemes hit over RMB1.22 trillion, covering about 30% of total health expenditure in China; the share of social insurance providers was less than 5% in 2001 (Figure 5-5).[20] The average upper limit for NCMS and URI amounted to six times of local average disposable income.[21] By the end of 2014, the reimbursement rates of BHI, URI and NCMS for inpatient services within the upper limit had reached 80%, 70% and 75% respectively.[22]

---

[20] *China Health Statistical Yearbook* and *China Labour and Social Security Yearbook,* various years.

[21] <http://www.gov.cn/hudong/2015-12/31/content_5058128.htm> (accessed 11 May 2016).

[22] Ministry of Human Resources and Social Security, Document no. 149, 2015, <http://www.mohrss.gov.cn/gkml/xxgk/201511/t20151120_226019.htm> (accessed 24 July 2016).

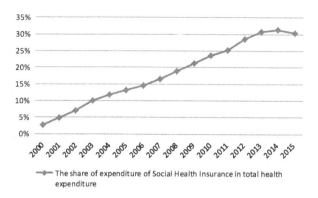

—◆— The share of expenditure of Social Health Insurance in total health expenditure

Figure 5-5: Amount of Reimbursement from Social Health Insurance as a Share of Total Health Expenditure
Source: *China Health Statistical Yearbook*, various years.

In March 2012, the State Council released a guideline for health reform between 2012 and 2015.[23] In June 2012, a guideline for social security reform for the 12th Five-Year Programme was jointly announced by six ministries.[24] Reform on social health insurance was covered by both guidelines. The coverage of social health plans will be universal and government will subsidise at least RMB360 per enrollee for NCMS and URI. Portability of social insurance within a province had been gradually implemented by 2015.[25] The development of private health insurance, as supplementary insurance, was also encouraged. Various payment methods, including capitation, "pay for performance", "global budget" and the Diagnosis Related Group (DRG),[26]

---

[23] <http://www.gov.cn/zwgk/2012-03/21/content_2096671.htm> (accessed 25 May 2016).
[24] <http://www.gov.cn/zwgk/2012-06/27/content_2171218.htm> (accessed 25 May 2016).
[25] <http://ghs.ndrc.gov.cn/zttp/xxczhjs/ghzc/201605/t20160520_802483.html> (accessed 25 July 2016).
[26] Capitation refers to the payment method in which a provider is reimbursed by insurers according to the number of enrollees treated by the provider. DRG is a

among others have been implemented on a larger scale. The role of purchaser (for social insurers) was highlighted in the negotiation of prices for health-care services.

Pilot projects for social insurance are being conducted in many localities. In Zhenjiang city, the pilot reform of payment method under social insurance plans has been used for hospitals. Payment methods for hospitals such as capitation and global budget have been adopted by social insurance plans in Zhenjiang city since 2001. In Henan province, global budget payment methods have been implemented for all rural NCMS enrollees.[27] Payment method reform has been carried out in county level hospitals in 311 counties nationwide from late 2012. In some of these pilots, traditional fee-for-service payment system has been replaced by various alternative payment methods to control cost within hospitals.[28]

In 2012, one interesting local pilot project in Guangzhou city, Guangdong province, allowed transferability of an individual's insurance card; family members were allowed to use the card,[29] which indirectly allowed risk pooling and increased financial coverage.

In July 2012, the State Council released a document called "Opinion on the establishment of supplementary health insurance for serious diseases".[30] According to this document, the objective of establishing supplementary insurance is to protect households from

---

payment method where the payment amount is determined by the type of diseases. Global budget refers to the payment method where a limit is placed on the total amount of money claimed by a provider. Pay for performance only allows reimbursement to be claimed by a provider after meeting certain performance measures for quality and efficiency.

[27] <http://news.xinhuanet.com/politics/2012-05/16/c_111964418.htm> (accessed 25 May 2016).

[28] <http://www.gov.cn/zwgk/2012-06/14/content_2161153.htm> (accessed 26 May 2016).

[29] <http://money.163.com/12/0515/18/81IM3BUG00253B0H.html> (accessed 26 May 2016).

[30] <http://finance.people.com.cn/insurance/n/2012/0831/c59941-18885344.html> (accessed 26 May 2016).

catastrophic health expenditure, a situation whereby households have to reduce their basic expenditure over a certain period to pay for health-care expenditure.[31] The establishment of supplementary insurance for NCMS and URI was also encouraged. For example, in Zhanjiang city, Guangdong province, the local government used 15% of NCMS/URI fund to buy private supplementary health insurance with a cap of RMB300,000. The local government of Chuxiong city, Yunnan province, encouraged its residents to buy supplementary private insurance (voluntarily) at a premium of RMB50 a year. NCMS and URI would cap at RMB60,000 instead of the previous RMB30,000.[32]

According to the 13th Five-Year Outline Plan for human resources and social security, by the end of 2020, reimbursement rate for inpatient service (i.e. regardless of the upper limit of insurance plans) is expected to reach 75%.[33] Two major directions of reform to achieve this goal have been considered in this plan. One is to consolidate insurance plans to increase risk pooling. The State Council has announced in November 2015 that in the future NCMS and URI in a city/prefecture would be merged into a single plan. In April 2016, the Ministry of Finance and Ministry of Human Resources and Social Security released a joint announcement that maternity insurance fund will be merged with health insurance fund (i.e. URI or BHI). The amount of accumulated surplus of the maternity insurance had reached over RMB57 billion in 2014, which may be helpful to improve the fiscal condition of health insurance.

The other direction of reform is the payment reform to increase the efficiency of the reimbursement from health insurance. In particular, the traditional fee-for-service payment system at county level

---

[31] <http://www.gov.cn/jrzg/2012-09/06/content_2217749.htm> (accessed 26 May 2016).
[32] <http://news.xinhuanet.com/fortune/2012-09/02/c_123661208.htm> (accessed 26 May 2016).
[33] *Beijing Evening News*, 15 July 2016, <http://bjwb.bjd.com.cn/html/2016-07/15/content_50355.htm> (accessed 7 October 2016).

hospitals in 311 counties nationwide from late 2012 would be replaced by various alternative payment methods to control cost in hospitals. By early 2016, over 85% and 35% of social insurance plans had implemented global budget and payment by standardised clinical paths respectively. In addition, 24% of insurance plans have implemented capitation.[34]

In the recent years, the payment method reform has become one of the major issues in the health reform. In Shanxi and Gansu provinces, DRG payment system is expected to be implemented on a large scale in 2016. In Sichuan, payment method reforms have been implemented in all public hospitals.[35]

Regulatory Issues for the Development of Social Health Insurance

One of the widely reported important regulatory issues is the abuse of reimbursement from social health insurance funds.[36] From the patient side, some enrollees were reported to have sold their insurance cards illegally to patients who are not covered by health insurance. In some other cases, some appointed drug sellers may even sell items outside of the eligible medicine list (including non-medical products) to obtain reimbursement.[37] More importantly, social insurance plans fail to control supplier-induced demand (i.e. physicians' opportunistic behaviours). Fee-for-service is still the major payment method between insurers and service providers. Alternative payment methods such as capitation and global budget are rarely used.

---

[34] For a detail discussion, see Chapter 6 of The World Bank Report, *Healthy China: Deepening Health Reform in China*, 2016, World Bank.

[35] <http://finance.people.com.cn/n1/2016/0524/c1004-28373383.html> (accessed 26 May 2016).

[36] <http://www.china.com.cn/news/txt/2010-11/02/content_21255111.htm> (accessed 26 May 2016).

[37] <http://finance.ifeng.com/insurance/bxlc/20120526/6520947.shtml> (accessed 26 May 2016).

In many cases, hospitals and patients have been reported to collude in claiming reimbursement from insurance funds.[38] Hospitals have incentives to provide unnecessary services to patients to claim reimbursement. With insurance coverage, patients are also willing to consume more health-care services (i.e. a moral hazard).

Financial sustainability of social insurance fund

Another very important regulatory issue in social insurance is the financial sustainability of social insurance funds. Contribution from urban workers' payroll and government subsidy are two major sources of the social insurance fund. The average annual growth rate of real wages was reportedly 13.8% between 1998 and 2010.[39] This implies that the contributions to social health insurance from urban labour would have correspondingly increased and at a very rapid speed. Likewise, government subsidy for social health insurance increased from RMB112.8 billion in 2008 to RMB565.7 billion in 2015.[40] Government subsidy for social health insurance accounted for over 41.8% of total government health expenditure in 2015 (Figure 5-6).

With the increasing number of enrollees, government subsidy for social insurance funds and urban wage rate, the surplus of social health insurance funds have expanded rapidly in recent years. Accumulated surplus of these three social health insurance plans accounted for more than 34% of health expenditure in 2015. Compared to the 10% of average surplus from international experiences, the surplus for all Chinese social health insurance is extremely high.

Fund surpluses have increased steadily in all three plans. Figures 5-7 shows the accumulated fund surpluses in BHI. Accumulated

---

[38] Liu Junqiang, et al., "Decomposing Health Inflation in China: An analysis based on historical data and field evidence", *Social Sciences in China*, no. 8, 2015, pp. 107–128.
[39] Li Hongbin, et al., "The End of Cheap Chinese Labor", *The Journal of Economic Perspectives*, vol. 26, no. 4, 2012, pp. 57–74.
[40] Budget Reports, Ministry of Finance, various years.

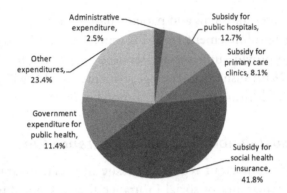

Figure 5-6: The Composition of Total Government Health Expenditure in 2015

Source: Budget Report 2016, Ministry of Finance.

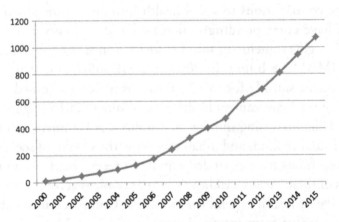

Figure 5-7: Fund Surplus for BHI (billion RMB)

Source: *China Labour and Social Security Yearbook*, various years.

surpluses for social pooling account in BHI increased by more than four times between 2004 and 2015 from RMB100 billion to about RMB1,073 billion (equivalent to over 145% of total reimbursement in 2015).[41] The accumulated fund surpluses for NCMS and URI

---

[41] Budget Report for social insurance funds, <http://sbs.mof.gov.cn/zhengwuxinxi/shujudongtai/201511/t20151116_1563903.html> (accessed 24 July 2016).

expanded from less than RMB19 billion in 2007 to over RMB438 billion in 2015 (i.e. 58.7% of total reimbursement in 2015).[42]

In particular, the surpluses of BHI and URI are significantly higher than the threshold level set by the Ministry of Finance in a guideline released in 2009. In that guideline, it was suggested that the surpluses in BHI's social pooling account be kept at between 50% and 75% of annual reimbursement. In 2015, the surpluses in URI and social pooling account of BHI combined reached RMB811.4 billion, accounting for about 108% of annual reimbursement in both plans, which are significantly higher than the 75% threshold.[43]

One important reason for these high surpluses in social health insurance is the relatively low financial coverage of these plans. Based on a recent audit report from a national audit report office,[44] the reimbursement rate for NCMS and URI (i.e. the ratio of reimbursed and health expenditure) were 49.2% and 52.3% respectively while the reimbursement rate of BHI were 64% in 2011. Simply put, out-of-pocket expenditures for enrollees under NCMS and URI account for about 50% of health expenses. For BHI, the out-of-pocket expenditure can still reach as high as 36% on average.

The high surpluses in some provinces are also attributable to the high contribution rate given the large number of migrants and relatively young age structure. For example, Guangdong is one of the major provinces receiving millions of migrant workers. While residents in Guangdong province only accounted for 7.8% of the population in China in 2014, surpluses of Guangdong's urban social insurance plans (i.e. BHI and URI) accounted for 14.6% of total surpluses nationwide

---

[42] Budget Report for social insurance funds, <http://sbs.mof.gov.cn/zhengwuxinxi/shujudongtai/201511/t20151116_1563903.html> (accessed 24 July 2016).
[43] Ministry of Human Resources and Social Security, *Statistical Communiqué on Human Resources and Social Security in China, 2015*, <http://www.mohrss.gov.cn/SYrlzyhshbzb/dongtaixinwen/buneiyaowen/201605/t20160530_240967.html> (accessed 21 December 2016).
[44] National Audit Office, Quanguo Shehui Baozhang jijin Shenji Jieguo, Announcement no. 34, 2012. <http://www.audit.gov.cn/n1992130/n1992150/n1992500/3071265.html> (accessed 18 May 2016).

in the same year.[45] In contrast, residents in Hebei, a northern province, accounted for 5.4% of population in China in 2014 and surpluses of urban social insurance accounted for only 3.9%.[46]

While surpluses are high currently, the financial sustainability is still a serious concern in the future. First, for some cities with an ageing population and shrinking industrial base, deficit in health insurance has emerged recently. In 2014, there were deficits in 185 of 380 BHI plans[47] (i.e. annual expenditure was more than contribution). In 2013, 22 BHI plans had exhausted all accumulated surpluses and 108 URI plans were in the red.[48] Cities with accumulated surpluses have decreased while those with deficits are on the rise.

Second, since almost everyone is covered by the social health insurance scheme, the premium revenue of health insurance funds is expected to increase at a slower rate. Meanwhile, since GDP growth in China has slowed, the growth rate of wages will be lower and so is the contribution to social insurance funds.

Third, expenditure from social health insurance is expected to increase significantly in the next five years. From the "13th Five-Year Outline Plan", the reimbursement rate for health expenditure will be increased significantly by 2020. For example, according to an Anhui province government announcement as reported by *Xinan Evening News*, the reimbursement rate for inpatient service is expected to increase for Anhui's NCMS to over 60% in 2016 from 58% in 2015. The reimbursement rate is thus expected to increase even further in the next five years.

While there are some initiatives in governance reform, inefficiency in the governance of hospitals and in the social health insurance scheme

---

[45] *China Labour and Social Security Yearbook.*

[46] *China Labour and Social Security Yearbook.*

[47] Zhu Hengpeng "Tuixiu zhigong shifou yinggai jiaofei canjia yibao", *Caixin*, 19 February 2016, <http://opinion.caixin.com/2016-02-19/100910741.html> (accessed 25 May 2016).

[48] *China Business Journal*, 27 June 2015, <http://news.sohu.com/20150627/n415733897.shtml> (accessed 25 May 2016).

is persistent. For example, in most cities/counties, there are three different types of social insurance plans managed by two different government agencies: local health bureau and social security bureau. Inefficiency is associated with the fragmented insurance system.[49] Currently over 100 million Chinese have reportedly joined more than one social health insurance plan and that over RMB20 billion subsidies have been issued to people who have enrolled in more than one social health insurance plan.[50] The inefficiency is in the issuance of subsidies to an enrollee more than once and in the various premiums paid by an enrollee to multiple health insurance plans when he or she can only be reimbursed by one insurance plan for health-care expenditure.

Capacity and Incentives of Social Insurers

Although social insurance schemes have improved greatly in China in the last recent decade, they have not fully functioned to implement reimbursement rules and improve on the financial conditions of social insurance fund. The incentives and capacity of social insurers are substantially relevant to addressing providers' profit-seeking behaviour. First, the incentive structure of social health insurance schemes is not compatible with the objective of the payment method reform. Many social health insurers' objective is merely to balance the budget and not to explore potential payment method reforms in order to control health service costs.[51] The future development of social insurance schemes is

---

[49] Meng Qingyue et al., "Consolidating the Social Health Insurance Schemes in China: Towards an equitable and efficient health system", *The Lancet*, vol. 386, 2015, pp. 1484–1492.

[50] <http://economy.caijing.com.cn/20140815/3658675.shtml> (accessed 4 August 2014).

[51] For example, a document released by Gaoan city of Jiangsu province in 2011 highlighted the importance of the balance in the insurance fund but not much was mentioned about the negotiation mechanism to reduce the treatment fee in the hospital. See <http://www.jxhrss.gov.cn/view.aspx?TaskNo=008&ID=105554> (accessed 4 August 2014) and Liu Junqiang, et al., "Decomposing Health Inflation in China: An analysis based on historical data and field evidence".

dependent on how the incentive of social insurers has been accommodated to induce them to work on the policy targets, such as choosing the most cost-effective treatment method as well as reducing the financial burden of the patients. Social health insurers, in general, have little incentive to improve the affordability of health-care services or to take full advantage of market mechanisms such as competition and purchasing to address the opportunistic behaviour of suppliers.

Local social insurers (local government) have the incentive to compete with other local governments since cadres' promotion prospects are highly dependent on their work performances.[52] When officials have multiple targets to fulfil, there is a tendency for them to pursue more measurable tasks such as accumulating more surpluses for insurance funds or promoting enrolment to social insurance plans. These tasks have greater visibility and are more rewarding for officials. In many counties, enrolment is usually reportedly inflated to meet targets set by the top leadership. In a city in Liaoning province, it is reported that the actual number of registrants to URI was only 27% of reported enrollees in 2011.[53]

One possible reason for accumulating an insurance fund surplus is the need to fulfil policy targets. For example, the Guangdong government plans to take advantage of its current fund surplus to buy reinsurance for a wider range of catastrophic health expenditure, which can extend insurance coverage beyond essential medicines and essential services.[54] Similar policies are implemented in Tianjin city and other cities including Ningbo city and Zhanjiang city.[55]

These governments use social insurance fund surpluses to promote the essential medicine system by subsidising service providers who

---

[52]Xu Chenggang, "The Fundamental Institutions of China's Reform and Development", *Journal of Economic Literature*, vol. 49, no. 4, 2011, pp. 1076–1151.

[53]*Daily Economic News* (Meiri Jinji Xingwen), 30 May 2012, <http://finance.sina.com.cn/china/20120530/011412175238.shtml> (accessed 25 May 2016).

[54]For a detailed discussion, please refer to Chapter 7 on the development of private health insurance.

[55]<http://finance.people.com.cn/GB/10915921.html> (accessed 25 May 2016).

suffered financial losses after price markups have been removed. Surplus of social insurance funds in Tianjin finances 9% out of the original 15% markup to encourage service providers to adopt the essential medicine system (the rest of the 6% is paid by fiscal budget). Such incentives (i.e. to divert surplus of social insurance fund for other arena of health reform) could be another explanation to the extraordinary amount of surplus that has been accumulated for social insurance.

To accumulate a surplus, the local government can either put a cap to the reimbursement for hospitals through negotiations and innovation of payment methods or simply keep the reimbursement rate at a relatively low level.[56] The first method may require more efforts on the part of the local government to conclude a contract by negotiation and bargaining.

Local government has strong incentive to set a relatively low reimbursement rate to balance the budget. Given the opportunistic behaviour of the insured and from supplier-induced demand, local insurers have the incentive to set a conservative reimbursement rate. According to a report by the National Audit Office in 2012,[57] the average reimbursement rate for many NCMS was around 50%. When treatment is done outside the county/city of registration, the reimbursement rate will be even lower (i.e. less than 30%).[58]

Second, though some localities have started pilot reforms of payment methods,[59] social insurers do not have the capacity/professional training to improve affordability via purchasing health services from

---

[56]Qian Jiwei and Ake Blomqvist, *Health Policy Reform in China* and Qian Jiwei, "Health Reform in China: Three years after", *EAI Background Brief*, no. 729, East Asian Institute, 14 June 2012.

[57]National Audit Office, Quanguo Shehui Baozhang jijin Shenji Jieguo, Announcement no. 34, 2012, <http://www.audit.gov.cn/n1992130/n1992150/n1992500/3071265.html> (accessed 18 May 2016).

[58]National Audit Office, Quanguo Shehui Baozhang jijin Shenji Jieguo.

[59]Cheng Tsung-Mei, "A Pilot Project Using Evidence-based Clinical Pathways and Payment Reform in China's Rural Hospitals Shows Early Success", *Health Affairs*, vol. 32, no. 5, 2013, pp. 963–973.

providers.[60] For example, there were about only 70 staff working in the social security bureau to manage over 19 million enrollees for social health insurance in Qingdao city in 2015. Compared to the international standard, the capacity is relatively low.[61]

Social health insurance schemes are also fragmentarily managed. Each prefecture should have at least three different plans (BHI, NCMS and URI). The administration cost is higher when these insurance programmes have to maintain their own health information system and invest in redundant information infrastructure. In January 2016, a new guideline was issued to integrate local NCMS and URI in coverage, financing and administration.[62] The coordination for the payment method reform is an issue since NCMS and URI were managed by two different bureaus: local health bureau and local social security bureau respectively. At the local level, small leading groups have been established to sort out the coordination issues. For example, in March 2016, Hunan province has initiated a small leading group for the consolidation of the social health insurance schemes.[63]

---

[60] Ramesh M, Wu Xun and Alex He Jingwei, "Health Governance and Health Care Reforms in China", *Health Policy and Planning*, vol. 29, 2013, pp. 663–72.

[61] *Jiankang Paper* (Jiankang Bao), 19 August 2015.

[62] <http://www.gov.cn/zhengce/content/2016-01/12/content_10582.htm> (accessed 13 May 2016).

[63] <http://epaper.hnmsw.com/view.asp?Aid=14608&Fid=5187> (accessed 26 May 2016).

Chapter 6

Medical Malpractice Dispute Resolution

Rise of Medical Malpractice Disputes

The increasing number of medical malpractice disputes is a serious concern in China.[1] Recent years have seen escalating tensions between patients and doctors, leading to a skyrocketing number of medical disputes and even violence.[2] In 2014, there were over 115,000 medical malpractice disputes in China.[3] According to the Chinese Hospital Management Association, the total number of disputes has been increasing by 22.9% a year since 2002.[4]

The lack of trust plays a significant role in the increasing disputes. A survey by *China Youth Daily* reported that nearly 70% of patients

[1] See Alex He Jingwei and Qian Jiwei, "Explaining Medical Disputes in Chinese Public Hospitals: The doctor-patient relationship and its implications for health policy reforms", *Health Economics, Policy and Law*, vol. 11, no. 4, 2016, pp. 359–378. See also doctor-patient relation and service quality in Chinese public hospitals in Qian Jiwei and Alex He Jingwei, "The Bonus Scheme, Motivation Crowding-Out and Quality of the Doctor-Patient Encounters in Chinese Public Hospitals", *Public Organization Review*, 2016.

[2] "Chinese Doctors Are under Threat" (editorial), *The Lancet*, vol. 376, Issue 9742, 2010, p. 657 and "Violence against Doctors: Why China? Why now? What next?" (editorial), *The Lancet*, vol. 383, Issue, 9922, 2014, p. 1013.

[3] <http://www.chinanews.com/gn/2015/01-22/6992666.shtml> (accessed 25 November 2016).

[4] <http://paper.people.com.cn/mszk/html/2014-03/10/content_1400738.htm> (accessed 25 May 2016).

do not trust physicians' diagnoses and treatments.[5] Another nationwide survey noted that only 26% of physicians felt that their patients trusted them and 70.9% would choose to pursue another occupation given the opportunity.[6]

Some of these disputes even ended up with violence towards doctors. On average, each Chinese hospital deals with 27 cases of violence targeted at doctors a year.[7] The total number of violent incidents against medical staff and hospitals had increased from 10,248 in 2006 to 17,243 in 2010, at a 13.9% annual growth rate.[8]

Regulatory policies and law enforcement are supposed to be very useful in this context. In principle, the regulator/court can enforce regulations/law to resolve a medical malpractice dispute if a doctor's negligent behaviour has been proven. Indeed, two regulations addressing medical malpractice disputes were released in 1987 and 2002 respectively. However, these two regulations were marred by the relatively low amount of compensation and uncertainty in enforcement due to their overlap with other regulations and laws, including the tort law, which has taken effect since 2010.[9] In November 2015, an amendment draft to malpractice dispute regulation was released by the

---

[5] *China Youth Daily* found that 87.6% of respondents expect to rebuild physician-patient trust, 22 November 2013, <http://zqb.cyol.com/html/2013-11/12/nw.D110000zgqnb_20131112_2-07.htm> (accessed 25 May 2016).

[6] *Life Daily*, "Mistrust between Doctors and Patients", 24 January 2014, <http://paper.people.com.cn/smsb/html/2014-01/24/content_1382292.htm> (accessed 23 July 2016.

[7] *Xinhua Daily Telegraph*, "Who Makes Doctors Sit on Top of Volcanoes?" 31 October 2013, <http://news.xinhuanet.com/mrdx/2013-10/31/c_132847265.htm> (accessed 25 May 2016).

[8] Feng Junmin, et al., "A Retrospective Analysis on 418 Medical Disputes", *Chinese Hospital Management*, vol. 33, Issue 9, 2013, pp. 77–79.

[9] Harris Dean and Wu Chien-Chang, "Medical Malpractice in the People's Republic of China: The 2002 regulation on the handling of medical accidents", *Journal of Law, Medicine and Ethics*, vol. 33, Issue 3, 2005, pp. 456–477 and Benjamin Liebman, "Malpractice Mobs: Medical dispute resolution in China".

National Health and Family Planning Commission.[10] The division of labour between malpractice dispute regulations and the tort law has been addressed in this amendment.

However, until recently, only a handful of patients employ litigation for resolution. In contrast to the sharp increase in disputes, the number of medical-related legal actions has only risen modestly even after the enactment of the Tort Liability Law in 2010.[11] For instance, only 19,944 lawsuits were reported in 2014, accounting for merely 17% of the total number of medical disputes recorded.[12]

The role of the regulator should thus be enhanced. An understanding of the institutional arrangements of the regulatory agencies and the incentives of the regulators is needed. This chapter discusses the institutional arrangement for malpractice dispute resolution. The performance evaluation system for local officials is one institutional reason for the ineffective enforcement of law and regulation. Like regulatory policy implementation in other areas of the Chinese health-care system, the "regulatory capture" in the context of public hospital governance is also a factor for the large number of violence in the hospitals. The choice of protests and violence[13] is a result of enforcement ineffectiveness. This chapter argues that future reforms may need to carefully address peculiarities in institutional arrangement and incentive structure of regulators.

---

[10]National Health and Family Planning Commission, "Notes about Drafting the Amendment of Malpractice Dispute Regulation", 2 November 2015. <http://www.nhfpc.gov.cn/zhuzhan/zcjd/201511/3b9643ca57004569ae44db8b967b49ba.shtml> (accessed 25 July 2016).

[11]Alex He Jingwei and Qian Jiwei, "Explaining Medical Disputes in Chinese Public Hospitals".

[12]NetEase News, 23 January 2016, <http://yd.sina.cn/article/detail-ifxnqrkc 6633526.d.html?oid=5_woai&vt=4&mid=cfkptvx3377037> (accessed 23 July 2016). Officially, 115,000 medical disputes were reported nationwide in 2014, <http://www.chinanews.com/gn/2015/01-22/6992666.shtml> (accessed 25 May 2016).

[13]Benjamin Liebman, "Malpractice Mobs: Medical dispute resolution in China".

Effectiveness of Resolution Mechanisms for Medical Malpractice Dispute

Medical malpractice refers to service providers' negligent behaviour leading to adverse events suffered by a patient. However, these adverse events may be the result of either the physician's behaviour or just an accident. This uncertainty may raise disputes of medical malpractice. The mechanism for resolving malpractice disputes is to achieve two objectives of compensating patients who have suffered from injury through negligence of health-care providers and deter service providers from further negligence, ex ante.[14]

However, it is very costly to write a contingency contract for malpractice ex ante since information on the treatment process is usually incomplete and fraught with uncertainties. Contracts are incomplete given these uncertainties and are not very useful to resolve disputes in this context.

From international experiences, regulations usually impose requirements ex ante and health service providers have to fulfil the criteria set by the regulator, failing which they will be punished regardless of whether the patients have suffered adverse effects or not. For example, US Food and Drug Administration (FDA) requires certain precautions to be fulfilled when dispensing drugs.

Litigation (i.e. filing a lawsuit against the hospital) and legally binding mediation are major mechanisms to resolve malpractice disputes for patients. Under the common law tradition, tort litigation is a mechanism satisfying both the aforementioned objectives to some extent: compensating patients and deterring negligent behaviours of doctors.[15] Patients can be compensated for negligent acts by practitioners ex post. Practitioners are deterred from wrong behaviour ex ante. However it is argued that the transaction cost for litigation in some

---

[14] Daniel Kessler, (ed.), *Regulation Versus Litigation: Perspectives from economics and law*, University of Chicago Press, 2011.

[15] Patricia Danzon, "Liability for Medical Malpractice", in Anthony Culyer and Joseph Newhouse (eds.), *Handbook of Health Economics*, vol. 1, 2000, pp. 1339–1404.

countries is so high that health expenditure has been driven upwards by defensive medicine used by doctors to reduce the probability of being sued by patients.[16] It was estimated that in the United States, the costs of defensive medicine together with other costs of medical liability system amounted to about US$55 billion in 2008.[17]

Mediation refers to "agreements between providers and patients to submit disputes over alleged malpractice to a third party other than a court". [18] The case can be settled at low cost and mediators may take advantage of informal and flexible solutions, depending on the context. Usually, the mediation is legally binding.[19]

Apart from the aforementioned major mechanisms, other private solutions relating to consensual, reciprocal, norms and so on are relevant. For example, guilds in medieval Europe played an important role in regulating compliance of traders with certain rules.[20]

In the context of China, regulatory policies for medical malpractice disputes have been implemented and they addressed both ex ante requirements as well as the rules for litigation. Two versions of regulations addressing medical accidents were released in 1987 and 2002 respectively. How litigation or administrative mediation can be processed has been considered in these two regulations. According to these two regulations, patients can only be compensated after a medical accident is identified through technical authentication to provide a professional judgement for the reasons of the malpractice.[21]

---

[16] Daniel Kessler, (ed.), *Regulation Versus Litigation*.

[17] Michelle Mello, et al., "National Costs of the Medical Liability System", *Health Affairs*, vol. 29, 9, 2010, pp. 1569–1577.

[18] Daniel P Kessler, "Evaluating the Medical Malpractice System and Options for Reform", *The Journal of Economic Perspectives*, vol. 25, no. 2, 2011, pp. 93–110.

[19] Daniel P Kessler, "Evaluating the Medical Malpractice System and Options for Reform".

[20] Avner Greif, Paul Milgrom and Barry R Weingast, "Coordination, Commitment, and Enforcement: The case of the merchant guild", *Journal of Political Economy*, vol. 102, no. 5 , 1994, pp. 745–776.

[21] Harris Dean and Wu Chien-Chang, *Medical Malpractice in the People's Republic of China*.

Besides these two regulations, other regulations have been imposed in Chinese hospitals including quality assurance, regulatory supervision and administrative discipline. Recently, tort litigation can be used in China when there are malpractice disputes. Tort Liability Law of the People's Republic of China has taken effect since July 2010. Under this recently released tort law, an authentication committee selected by the local health bureau was still the major body for reviewing the negligent behaviour of service providers. The negligence principle has been used in malpractice cases in China after 2002.

Patients can also use administrative mediation to resolve disputes. Local health bureaus are usually considered as the administrative mediator. Authentication process is also required for administrative mediation. Administrative mediation is considered to be legally binding.[22]

However, in some recent research and reports, a significant proportion of patients prefer protests to litigation and administrative mediation to resolve the disputes.[23] According to a survey by China Hospital Association in 316 hospitals, in 2012, violent incidents resulting in significant injuries of doctors or nurses in 63.7% of public hospitals, increased from 47.7% in 2008.[24]

In Nanjing, Jiangsu, 90% of medical disputes ended up in violence. In Guangdong, it was reported that there was an average of one incident of violence against hospitals a day in 2006.[25] From interviews in a municipality, it was reported that violence is "common" and local hospital officials and their lawyers complain that "police are slow or unwilling to respond".[26]

---

[22] See The State Council, "Regulation on the Implementation of the Administrative Reconsideration Law of the People's Republic of China", 2007, <http://www.gov.cn/zwgk/2007-06/08/content_641675.htm> (accessed 11 August 2016).
[23] Wu Weiqing and Jing Yifeng, "Analysis of Patients' Behaviors, Attitudes, and Complaints in Medical Disputes", *Chinese Medical Ethics*, 2010, pp. 24–25 and Benjamin Liebman, "Malpractice Mobs: Medical dispute resolution in China".
[24] <http://www.chinanews.com/fz/2014/01-27/5786914.shtml> (accessed 11 May 2016).
[25] Benjamin Liebman, "Malpractice Mobs: Medical dispute resolution in China".
[26] Benjamin Liebman, "Malpractice Mobs: Medical dispute resolution in China".

The under-utilisation of authentication

The stagnant number of technical authentication cases shows the under-utilisation of major resolution mechanisms such as litigation and administrative mediation as technical authentication is required for these mechanisms. According to the 2002 regulation about medical accidents, authentication can be conducted at municipal level or provincial level.[27] The number of authentication cases, reported by the China Medical Association, has not increased and even decreased since 2004 while the number of medical malpractice disputes has increased by over 20% annually since 2002 (Table 6-1).

Ineffectiveness of Regulation Enforcement: Incentives and Institutions

This section argues that the incentive structure of bureaucrats is subject to a couple of institutional constraints, namely, performance evaluation

Table 6-1:   Number of Authentication Cases in China[28]

Year	Municipal Level Cases	Provincial Level Cases	Total
2003	6,700	1,600	8,300
2004	9,089	2,943	12,032
2005	9,714	2,396	12,110
2006	10,184	2,338	12,522
2007	10,207	2,373	12,580
2008	10,929	2,563	12,492
2010	10,479	2,488	12,967
2012	8,859	2,215	11,144
2013	8,604	2,140	10,744

Source: China Medical Association.

[27] <http://www.people.com.cn/GB/shenghuo/76/123/20020415/709626.html> (accessed 25 July 2016).
[28] 2009 and 2011 data are missing. See <http://www.cma.org.cn/bainian/zhuanti/2015325/1427270827701_1.html> (accessed 25 July 2016).

system and organisational arrangement for policy implementation. Bureaucrats then enforce law and regulations to meet their best interests. The incentives of the bureaucrats and relevant institutional arrangements such as governance structure of public hospitals result in the rise in protest against medical malpractice.

Bureaucrats' behaviour in China decides law and regulation enforcement in two ways. First, the regulations set by bureaucrats and literature show that public policy is a product of bureaucratic bargaining in China.[29] Compared to bureaucrats in Mao's era, bureaucrats now are even more influential and have the incentives to pursue their own goals strategically in the process of policy implementation. Second, bureaucrats have discretion over policy implementation and law enforcement. Unlike regulatory entities in many other countries where regulatory agencies are institutionally separated from the ordinary bureaucracy and politicians to avoid a conflict of interest,[30] "the executive branch has predominated in the formulation and implementation of regulatory laws and policies" in China.[31] Recent research also shows that local governments have discretion over judicial decisions.[32]

The ineffectiveness of regulation and law enforcement is thus closely associated with the incentives of bureaucrats, chiefly, the performance evaluation system for government officials and the organisation arrangements for enforcing the laws. The former is the main institutional cause for the weak enforcement of regulations while the latter are

---

[29] Kenneth G Lieberthal and Michel Oksenberg, *Policy Making in China: Leaders, structures, and processes*, Princeton, Princeton University Press, 1988, p. 4.

[30] Gilardi Fabrizio and Martino Maggetti, "The Independence of Regulatory Authorities", in David Levi-Faur (ed.), *Handbook on the Politics of Regulation*, Cheltenham, Edward Elgar, 2011, pp. 201–214.

[31] Tam Waikeung and Yang Dali, "Food Safety and the Development of Regulatory Institutions in China", *Asian Perspective*, vol. 29, no. 4, 2005, pp. 5–36.

[32] Lee Ching Kwan and Zhang Yonghong, "The Power of Instability: Unraveling the microfoundations of bargained authoritarianism in China", *American Journal of Sociology*, vol. 118, no. 6, 2013, pp. 1475–1508 and Su Yang and He Xin, "Street as Courtroom: State accommodation of labor protest in South China", *Law and Society Review*, vol. 44, Issue 1, 2010, pp. 157–84.

the "regulatory capture" (i.e. regulators representing the interests of the regulated); "regulatory capture" is closely associated with the governance structure of public hospitals in the context of the medical malpractice disputes.

Medical malpractice dispute and performance evaluation system

The introduction chapter discusses the importance of fiscal revenue and GDP growth for evaluating local officials. Of equal importance is social stability, a criterion in an official's performance evaluation system which has veto power for his or her promotion or appointment.[33] In other words, if there is any incident such as protests, local officials may not be able to be promoted or appointed. For local officials, social stability is usually positively correlated to the success rate of mediation and negatively correlated to the number of collective incidences (*qunti xin shijian*) where stakeholders do not accept mediation. There is strong incentive then for local governments to discourage conflict/collective incidence and encourage hospitals and patients to reach a successful settlement.

Local governments are not only stakeholders but also enforcers of regulations related to these violent incidents in hospitals. From recent research, local bureaucrats prefer mediation to litigation since mediation is an immediate solution to resolve disputes.[34] When the scale and intensity of violence grows and "social stability" may be affected, local governments have strong incentive to seek to pacify patients even when violence had been used against hospital staff. Simply put, local

---

[33] The satisfaction of five criteria will grant veto power to local officials in their promotion: social stability, family planning, anti-corruption, work safety, and letters and visits (to upper level government). Officials will not be promoted when they fail to fulfil any one of these indexes See <http://www.chinanews.com/gn/2011/12-09/3521290.shtml> (accessed 11 May 2015). For a more detailed discussion, see Wang Yuhua, *Tying the Autocrat's Hands*.

[34] Lee Ching Kwan and Zhang Yonghong, *The Power of Instability: Unraveling the microfoundations of bargained authoritarianism in China*.

governments may selectively enforce the law or regulation to resolve the disputes, on the basis of the scale/intensity of the violence. It was also observed that judicial decision is not often made independently. Rather, many judicial decisions are made subject to local governments' incentives.[35]

Aware of the importance of social stability to local government's promotion, patients may capitalise on this fact and mobilise resources and place their demands in the form of violence or protests. The government is likely to use different strategies depending on its assessment of patients' capacity for mobilising resources. The resource capacity of patients may depend on the strength of local connection, income level and so on.

Medical malpractice dispute and public hospital governance

For resolving medical malpractice disputes, the authentication process matters greatly as medical professionals will have to justify whether the hospital/doctor should be liable arising out of the medical malpractice dispute. However, the authentication process is often not very credible, propelling people to protest and resort to violence.

Patients are aware of the existence of "regulatory capture" in the authentication process where decision makers in the authentication represent the interests of doctors, given the governance structure of public hospitals.

Public hospitals were dominant in the health service market in China and accounted for over 90% of hospital revenue and over 85% of inpatient service volume in 2015.[36] Under the current Chinese legal system, public hospitals rather than individual doctors are the ones responsible for the medical malpractice.[37]

---

[35] For example, see Lee Ching Kwan and Zhang Yonghong, *The Power of Instability* and Su Yang and He Xin, "Street as Courtroom".

[36] *China Health and Family Planning Statistical Yearbook*, 2016.

[37] Harris Dean and Wu Chien-Chang, *Medical Malpractice in the People's Republic of China*. Jordan Kearney, "Why China's 2010 Medical Malpractice Reform Fails to

Public hospitals are managed by the local health bureau and controlled by local governments to a significant degree.[38] Many officials in the local health bureaus were formally medical doctors and local health bureau and public hospitals are therefore closely connected by the personnel and administrative ties. The twin role of the local health bureau, as the manager of local public hospitals and coordinator of the authentication process, implies that local health bureau is both the regulator and regulated (given that public hospitals are liable for malpractice), a similar situation as the "regulator capture" in medical malpractice disputes.

In this context, the authentication process required in the major dispute resolution mechanisms including litigation and administrative mediation is not very credible for two reasons. Firstly, the authentication process lacks transparency in the selection of the authentication committee member. Local health bureau picks committee member from local hospital doctors who may not adopt an independent stance especially if the defendant of an investigation is also a public hospital doctor in the same locality.

Secondly, an authentication committee member is not required to endorse or write a testimony for the case investigated. This arrangement puts doubt on the credibility of the authentication process. The local health bureau, as a regulator, is believed to be likely to represent the interests of public hospitals.

The governance mode of public hospitals is also why many patients use violence in disputes pertaining to malpractice. As local governments would prefer to settle disputes at a non-legal level, many forced public hospitals to make compensations as public hospitals are not independent from the government.[39] Even after the recent round of public hospital reform, local governments still have the capacity to influence public hospitals through personnel appointment and other avenues.

Reform Medical Malpractice", *Emory International Law Review*, vol. 26, Issue 2, 2012, pp. 1039–1078.
[38] Jordan Kearney, "Why China's 2010 Medical Malpractice Reform Fails to Reform Medical Malpractice".
[39] Qian Jiwei and Ake Blomqvist, *Health Policy Reform in China.*

Alternative Dispute Resolution Mechanisms

To resolve disputes, alternative mechanisms other than litigation and administrative mediation have been considered. For example, a new initiative that involves people's mediation (*renmin tiaojie*) has been promoted in China recently to respond to protests and violent incidents in hospitals. Patients could solicit consultants in this type of mediation. Mediators consist of retired professionals including retired lawyers and doctors. These mediators are paid by the government. People's mediation is said to have more credibility than administrative mediation because local justice bureau rather than health bureau has been put in charge.

Compared to other mechanisms, costs for people's mediation are lower and settlement could be reached earlier. Unlike major dispute resolution mechanisms including litigation and administrative mediation, no authentication is required for people's mediation, which may increase the creditability of the process. Besides, the decisions made under people's mediation are not legally binding.

People's mediation has reportedly been used in 73.8% of counties by October 2011, processing over 14,000 disputes. By end 2012, people's mediation had covered every county in China. In 2015, about 71,000 medical malpractice disputes utilised people's mediation nationwide, settling over 85% of these cases.[40]

Insurance schemes have also played an important role in people's mediation. In a document released in August 2014, National Health and Family Planning Commission, together with other four ministries, has highlighted the role of medical liability insurance in the dispute resolution, in particular its role in supporting people's mediation.[41] If a hospital participates in the medical liability insurance scheme (*yiliao zeren xian*), insurance companies will reimburse the hospitals some of

---

[40] *Legal Daily*, 25 February 2016, <http://www.moj.gov.cn/jcgzzds/content/2016-02/25/content_6497390.htm?node=405> (accessed 11 August 2016).

[41] <http://www.nhfpc.gov.cn/yzygj/s3589/201407/65d55251804c408581a4e58db4 1f4bc7.shtml> and <http://finance.ce.cn/rolling/201608/12/t20160812_14787570. shtml> (accessed 11 May 2016).

the compensation paid to patients to settle the disputes. By the end of 2015, all major public hospitals in urban China were participants of the medical liability insurance scheme.[42] In 2015, the premium revenue for the medical liability insurance scheme reached RMB2.3 billion, an over 25% increase from that of 2014.[43] Reimbursement from insurance reached RMB1.4 billion.[44]

The institutional constraints and incentive structure of regulators under the resolution mechanism such as litigation and administrative mediation have made people's mediation a viable community level governance mechanism based on local knowledge and social norms rather than rule of law. In a broader context, community level governance mechanism can be a substitute or a complement to public enforcement mechanism,[45] depending on which stage of development the community is in.[46]

Recent studies show that a higher proportion of cases have been solved by alternative dispute resolution mechanisms such as people's mediation rather than through formal mechanisms including litigation and administrative mediation.[47] In the amendment draft to malpractice

---

[42] <http://china.caixin.com/2016-03-28/100925607.html> (accessed 11 August 2016).

[43] <http://china.caixin.com/2016-03-28/100925607.html> (accessed 11 August 2016).

[44] <http://china.caixin.com/2016-03-28/100925607.html> (accessed 11 August 2016).

[45] Mitchell A Polinsky and Steven Shavell, "The Theory of Public Enforcement of Law", in *Handbook of Law and Economics*, Elsevier, 2007.

[46] Scott Masten and Jens Prüfer, "On the Evolution of Collective Enforcement Institutions: Communities and courts", *Journal of Legal Studies*, vol. 43, no. 2, 2014, pp. 359-400.

[47] Only a handful of disputes were reported to have been solved by litigation from a hospital survey reported in Alex He Jingwei and Qian Jiwei, "Explaining Medical Disputes in Chinese Public Hospitals". For a study in a broader context, see Tang Wenfang, *Populist Authoritarianism: Chinese political culture and regime sustainability*, Oxford, Oxford University Press, 2015, which argues that most of the labour disputes have been resolved by alternative resolution mechanisms other than formal

dispute regulation released in November 2015, formal regulations for people's mediation were being considered[48] as local governments have devised their own regulations pertaining to people's mediation in recent years.[49]

However, the resolution of a dispute under people's mediation is not legally binding. The decision made by people's mediation is specific to that particular context and such a case cannot be used as a binding precedent for other cases or in other localities. It is less likely that this kind of alternative governance mode could develop into a viable system for resolving disputes in a sustainable way as it involves considerable externalities across communities (e.g. in the arena of public health and dispute resolution mechanism). In the country's transition to a market economy, the regulatory system has to be formal and impersonal, and to substitute the informal institutions.[50] It is thus unlikely that people's mediation will become the major resolution mechanism for medical malpractice disputes. Reforming the institutional arrangements, such as amending the performance evaluation system of officials, reforming the governance mode of public hospitals and adjusting the requirements for the authentication process, is hence necessary.

---

mechanisms. Interestingly, in Wang Yuhua, *Tying the Autocrat's Hands*, compared to foreign-owned firms, private and state-owned firms are more likely to use mediation than litigation to resolve disputes.

[48] <http://www.nhfpc.gov.cn/zhuzhan/zcjd/201511/3b9643ca57004569ae44db8b9 67b49ba.shtml> (accessed 25 July 2016).

[49] For example, in Fujian, a regulation on resolving medical malpractice disputes have been enacted since July 2016 and people's mediation, according to this regulation, plays a significant role in resolving malpractice disputes. See <http://www.fujian.gov. cn/zc/zwgk/flfg/zfgz/201606/t20160602_1174746.htm> (accessed 10 August 2016).

[50] For a similar argument for the accountability and development of impersonal rule in China, see Barry Naughton, "Inside and Outside: The modernized hierarchy that runs China", *Journal of Comparative Economics*, vol. 44, Issue 2, 2016, pp. 404–415.

Chapter 7

The Emerging Private Sector in the Chinese Health-care System

Regulation and the Role of the Private Sector in the Chinese Health-care System

As what has been discussed in Chapter 2, it is always one of the top priorities of the Chinese government to make Chinese health care affordable and accessible. This is reflected in the upward trend of health expenditure. Total health expenditure reached RMB4 trillion, or about 6% of GDP in 2015,[1] while the annual growth rate of out-of-pocket expenditure between 2008 and 2015 was a high of 11%.

The demand for health service has also shown an upswing, with the annual number of visits to tertiary hospitals increasing by over 840 million between 2009 and 2015.[2] Hospitals could hardly meet the demand. Bed utilisation rate in tertiary hospitals (*"sanji yiyuan"*) has been over 100% since 2009.

---

[1] National Health and Family Planning Commission, *Statistical Communiqué of Health and Family Planning in China, 2015*, <http://www.nhfpc.gov.cn/guihuaxxs/s10748/201607/da7575d64fa04670b5f375c87b6229b0.shtml> (accessed 24 July 2016).

[2] National Health and Family Planning Commission, *Statistical Communiqué of Health and Family Planning in China, 2015* and *China Health Statistical Yearbooks*, various years.

There is thus great potential for the private sector to explore this growing market and to fill the shortfall. With the entry of the private sector in the health-care service sector, prices of services and drugs will be more competitive and affordability of health care could be improved.

So is the accessibility of health care. The entry of the private sector in health insurance could also help expand the financial coverage of patients by reimbursing a wider range of services. Private health insurance would also be useful in raising the limit of the financial coverage of social health insurance. There are also over 100 companies offering private insurance products. Annual premium revenue registered over RMB240 billion in 2015.[3]

The significance of the private sector in health-care service market has also grown. In 2015, a 22% of outpatient services were provided by privately owned providers and private hospitals accounted for about 15% of inpatient services among all hospitals.[4]

However, there is still much room for the private sector to grow in health-care service delivery and health insurance in China. The scale of private hospitals is still small. In 2015, only 174 private hospitals versus more than 2,880 public hospitals had more than 500 beds. In terms of service efficiency, private hospitals are clearly lagging behind.

Private insurance is also underdeveloped, to some degree. While the amount of premium of private insurance had increased to over RMB110 billion in 2013, the ratio of premium revenue and total health expenditure witnessed a slight dip to 3.5%, from 3.67% in 2003. Products of private insurance agencies could not attract consumers in particular after the expansion of social health insurance in 2009. Between 2013 and 2015, private health insurance experienced a rapid increase. In 2015, the ratio of premium revenue and total health

---

[3] <http://www.circ.gov.cn/web/site0/tab5257/info4014824.htm> (accessed 24 December 2016).
[4] National Health and Family Planning Commission, *Statistical Communiqué of Health and Family Planning in China, 2015*.

expenditure increased to 5.9%.[5] However the ratio is still low compared to other countries, such as the 35% of the United States, about 10% of France and about 10% of Canada.[6]

In this context, the regulatory system is needed to ensure the quality of health-care services and health insurance plans. However, the current underdevelopment of the private sector could be attributed to some issues of the regulatory systems which may include strict regulations for the private sector actors, insurance designation bias against private hospitals and low capacity in enforcing regulation.

In the official document of the Third Plenum of the 18th Party Congress released in November 2013, the entry of the private sector in the health-care service market is encouraged.[7] Some concrete policies including deregulation of the health service market and public-private collaboration in the health insurance sector have been introduced.

In October 2014, the State Council announced a government action plan to promote private health insurance.[8] In January 2015, the State Council endorsed a guideline for health resource planning for the period 2015–2020.[9] The establishment of private hospitals and hospitals with mixed ownership has been encouraged in this guideline.

Another policy guideline for regulating the practices of doctors was released by the National Health and Family Planning Commission in January 2015.[10] This policy is to promote the mobility of doctors so as to fill the shortage of medical practitioners in the private sector.

---

[5] <http://www.circ.gov.cn/web/site0/tab5205/info4014828.htm> (accessed 24 July 2016).
[6] <https://www.oecd.org/health/health-systems/Focus-Health-Spending-2015.pdf> (accessed 24 July 2016).
[7] <http://news.xinhuanet.com/politics/2013-11/15/c_118164235.htm> (accessed 28 February 2015).
[8] <http://www.gov.cn/zhengce/content/2014-11/17/content_9210.htm> (accessed 28 February 2015).
[9] <http://finance.sina.com.cn/chanjing/cyxw/20150120/011921334930.shtml> (accessed 28 February 2015).
[10] <http://www.nhfpc.gov.cn/yzygj/s3577/201501/8663861edc7d40db91810ebf0ab996df.shtml> (accessed 28 February 2015).

In the recent years, the entry of the private sector in the health service market took two forms. One is privatisation of public hospitals. The other is the restructuring of hospitals' capital structure into the form of a mixed ownership. In terms of health insurance, private insurers have been introduced to complement the social health insurance "catastrophic medical insurance programme" to improve the financial coverage of patients.

Despite the efforts made, institutional constraints for the development of the private sector remain after the recent regulatory reform. The deregulation of private hospitals is still at an early stage, while the strict regulation of private insurers and the absence of a tax rebate policy for private insurance prevail.

The Role of the Private Sector in Improving Affordability and Accessibility

In its eighth year of implementation, China's most recent set of health reforms has yet to fully achieve its objectives of building a health system that will be accessible to and affordable for all Chinese citizens by 2020.

Health expenditure remains on the high side. Particularly for rural residents, out-of-pocket health expenditure accounted for 9.2% of total household expenditure in 2015 compared to 7.2% in 2009.[11] Out-of-pocket health expenditure amounted to over RMB1.25 trillion in 2015, while the annual growth rate of out-of-pocket expenditure between 2008 and 2015 reached 11%.[12]

Accessibility is another important issue for the Chinese health-care system. The demand for health-care services has increased rapidly and it is increasingly difficult for hospitals to meet the demand given their capacity. Figure 7-1 shows that the workload of a doctor in a tertiary hospital had increased by over 13.5% between 2009 and 2014. In 2015, doctors' workload had reduced slightly for all levels of hospitals. Bed utilisation rate had shown a marked increase for all levels

---

[11] *China Health and Family Planning Statistical Yearbook 2016.*
[12] See Chapter 2.

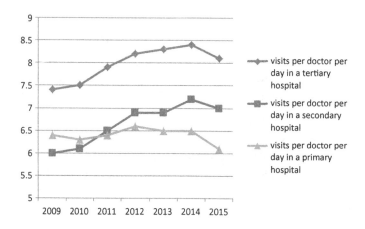

Figure 7-1: Visits Per Doctor Per Day for Different Levels of Hospitals.
Source: *China Health Statistical Yearbook*, various years and *Statistical Communiqué on Health and Family Planning in China, 2015.*

of hospitals between 2008 and 2014, particularly for tertiary hospitals where the bed utilisation rate was well over 100%.

Given the rapid rise in demand for health-care services, the Chinese government is looking at the private sector to boost accessibility and affordability of health care. Accessibility will be enhanced with more health-care service providers in the market. Patients could look forward to more affordable health-care services particularly for drugs with the entry of the private sector and the increased competition.

Private insurers can also play a role in improving affordability by complementing or supplementing public health insurance.[13] Private insurance schemes can either cover the co-payment part and increasing the upper limit of reimbursement (i.e. complementary private insurance) or services/drugs not covered by the public plan (i.e. supplementary private insurance).

---

[13] Usage of the terms "substitute private insurance", "complementary private insurance" and "supplementary private insurance" follows OECD terminology. See Colombo, Francesca and Nicole Tapay, "Private Health Insurance in OECD Countries: The benefits and costs for individuals and health systems", *OECD Health Working Papers*, no. 15, 2004.

In the Chinese context, given a relatively "low" upper limit of insurance coverage and many regulated services and drugs[14] under social health insurance, complementary and supplementary private insurance is particularly useful for covering non-basic services/essential drugs and increasing the coverage of insurance schemes.

Private insurance schemes with considerable bargaining power may discipline health service providers to reduce physician-induced demand through contractual arrangements on treatment procedures and prices.

Private insurers can also provide management expertise for social insurers. While some localities have started pilot reforms of payment methods to improve financial coverage,[15] social insurers do not have the capacity or the professional training to improve affordability by negotiating and purchasing health services from providers.[16]

Underdevelopment of Private Hospitals and Private Health Insurance Schemes

The private sector is gaining importance in the Chinese health-care system as evidenced by the voluminous growth in outpatient visits to privately owned hospitals from 66 million in 2005 to over 370 million in 2015.[17] The share of hospitals in total outpatient visits to hospitals surged from 8% in 2009 to 12% in 2015 (Figure 7-2). However, Figure 7-2 also shows that the share of outpatient volume for all privately owned service providers (including private hospitals and other privately owned primary care clinics) had decreased from 23.7% in 2011 to 22.3% in 2015.

---

[14]These regulated services and drugs refer to basic health-care services and essential medicines.

[15]Cheng Tsung-Mei, "A Pilot Project Using Evidence-Based Clinical Pathways and Payment Reform in China's Rural Hospitals Shows Early Success", *Health Affairs*, vol. 32, no. 5, 2012, pp. 963–973.

[16]Ramesh M, Wu Xun and Alex He Jingwei, "Health Governance and Health Care Reforms in China".

[17]*Statistical Communiqué on Health and Family Planning in China, 2015*.

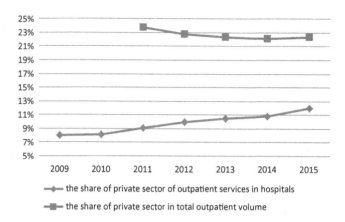

Figure 7-2:   Outpatient Visits to Privately Owned Services Providers[18]

Source: Statistical Communiqué on Health and Family Planning in China, various years.

Inpatient services provided by private hospitals also saw phenomenal increase from two million in 2005 to about 23.7 million in 2015. The share of private hospitals in inpatient services provided by all hospitals increased from 4% in 2005 to 14.7% in 2015 (Figure 7-3).

The turnover of private insurance agencies has also registered rapid expansion. The premium revenue of private insurance in 2015 reached RMB241 billion, with a 36% annual growth since 2011.[19] There were over 100 companies offering private health insurance and about 2,300 private insurance products were offered in the market in 2014.[20]

However, both private hospitals and private insurance are underdeveloped. First, the scale of private hospitals is relatively small, implying that many private health service providers lack the capacity to meet the growing demand.

---

[18] The data for outpatient service volume in privately owned providers before 2011 is missing.

[19] <http://www.circ.gov.cn/web/site0/tab5257/info4014824.htm> (accessed 28 December 2016).

[20] <http://scitech.people.com.cn/n/2015/0227/c1057-26602601.html> (accessed 12 March 2015).

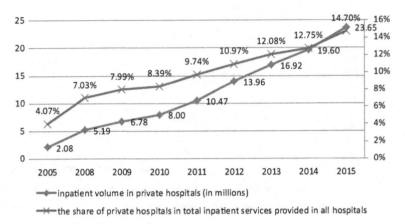

Figure 7-3: Inpatient Visits to Privately Owned Hospitals

Source: *China Health Statistical Yearbook*, various years and *Statistical Communiqué on Health and Family Planning in China, 2015.*

Table 7-1: Number of Public and Private Hospitals by Their Capacity in 2015

	Total	0–49	50–99	100–199	200–299	300–399	400–499	500–799	800 and above
Public	13,069	2,989	1,730	2,265	1,389	1,009	801	1,452	1,434
Private	14,518	6,814	3,668	1,808	456	179	58	116	58

Source: *China Health and Family Planning Statistical Yearbook*, various years.

Table 7-1 shows that though the number of private hospitals is considerable, most of the hospitals are small in size. In 2015, about 170 private hospitals versus more than 2,800 public hospitals had more than 500 beds. About 48% of private hospitals had more than 50 beds while more than 77% of public hospitals had more than 50 beds.

In terms of service provision, the utilisation rate in public hospitals is much higher than the utilisation rate of private hospitals. In 2015, the utilisation rates of public and private hospitals on average were 90% and 63% respectively (Figure 7-4).

The development of private insurance is also not as fast as expected in the recent decade. While the amount of premium of private

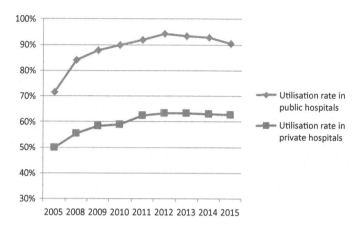

Figure 7-4:   Bed Utilisation Rate in Public and Private Hospitals

Source: *China Health Statistical Yearbook*, various years and *Statistical Communiqué on Health and Family Planning in China, 2015.*

insurance had increased to over RMB110 billion in 2013, the ratio of premium and health expenditure was only about 3.5%, a slight dip compared to 3.67% in 2003 (Figure 7-5). Between 2013 and 2015, the premium from private health insurance had increased very rapidly; in 2015, the ratio of premium and health expenditure increased to 5.94%.

Compared to other countries, private health insurance is relatively underdeveloped in China. The amount of reimbursement from private insurance only accounted for 1.3% of total health expenditure in 2013, while the ratio was over 10% each in Germany, France, the United States and Canada.[21]

Products introduced by private insurance agencies also lack appeal particularly after the expansion of social health insurance. In 2003, private health insurance enjoyed the patronage of 9.4% of households in China. However, after social health insurance has been expanded in

---

[21] <http://finance.chinanews.com/fortune/2015/02-25/7076607.shtml> (accessed 26 February 2015).

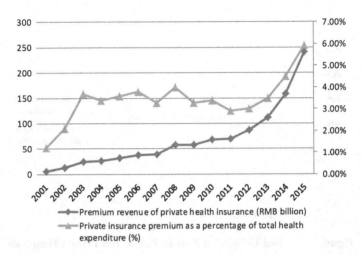

Figure 7-5: Premium of Private Health Insurance and Share of Premium in Total Health Expenditure

Source: *China Health Statistical Yearbook*, various years.

urban and rural areas, only a respective 6.9% and 6.3% of households in 2008 and 2010 had private health insurance.[22]

Institutional Constraints to the Development of the Private Sector

Constraints for the entry of private sector in the health service market and health insurance market are aplenty. First, regional health resource plan, which is formulated by the local health authority, has imposed restrictions on new entrants in the health-care service sector.[23]

The plan also seemingly favours public hospitals in terms of the quota set for the number of providers, hospital beds, human resources

---

[22] Yan Xiaolin, et al., "Commercial Health Insurance under the New Healthcare Reform: Status, problems and strategies", *China Journal of Health Policy*, vol. 6, no. 5, 2013, pp. 50–54.

[23] *Chongqing Daily*, 31 October 2014, <http://cq.ce.cn/syc/roll/201410/31/t20141031_1868806.shtml> (accessed 26 February 2015).

and equipment.[24] Other regulatory constraints over land use, tax rebate, among others also prevail.

Second, doctors of private hospitals lack professional recognition in terms of the granting of professional rank, research projects and participation in academic activities and others. Most doctors in private hospitals are either retirees from public hospitals or fresh graduates. There are very few experienced doctors. For example, a recent report shows that in a private hospital in Chongqing, 30% of the employees were retirees and recent graduates accounted for another 60%.[25]

Third, the status of (social) insurance designated hospital is important for private hospitals given the universal coverage of social health insurance.[26] However, private hospitals face restrictions in obtaining such designation particularly imposed by rural social health insurance due to the regulation set by the local health and social insurance authority.[27] Even for private hospitals with such designation, the insurance policy is different from that of public hospitals.[28]

Fourth, the lack of bargaining power has put private health insurers at risk as they could not negotiate for the desired payment method with public hospitals. Profitability is hence low for private health insurers. Over 40% of private health insurers are reported to have reimbursed more than 100% of their premium income, with some reimbursing even more than 200% of their premium income to patients.[29]

---

[24] See Chapter 1 of Chen Peifu and Wang Peizhou, *Development Report on Private Hospitals in China* ("Minyin Yiyuan Lanpi Shu: Zhongguo Minyin Yiyuan Fazhan Baogao") (1984–2012), Beijing, Social Sciences Academic Press, 2013.

[25] <http://www.lwgcw.com/NewsShow.aspx?newsId=34972> (accessed 26 February 2015).

[26] Alex He Jingwei, "Developing the Private Medical Sector in China", *EAI Background Brief*, no. 921, East Asian Institute, National University of Singapore, 22 May 2014.

[27] See Chapter 1 of Chen Peifu and Wang Peizhou, *Development Report on Private Hospitals in China*.

[28] <http://www.china.com.cn/chinese/health/zhuanti/ylws/1231432.htm> (accessed 26 February 2015).

[29] Yan Xiaolin, et al., "Commercial Health Insurance under the New Healthcare Reform".

Fifth, the expansion and increasing financial coverage of social health insurance has imposed a crowding out effect on private health insurance. Fewer households have registered with private insurers after the expansion of social health insurance since the mid 2000s.[30]

Health Reform and New Government Initiatives

The entry of the private sector in the health-care service market has been encouraged in the official document of the Third Plenum of the 18th Party Congress released in November 2013.[31] The government has since released a number of documents delineating the role of the private sector.

In December 2013, a series of policies were announced to encourage private sector participation.[32] First, hospitals with Hong Kong, Taiwan and Macau investors are allowed to operate in prefecture-level cities, while those controlled by investors of other foreign countries can operate in the Shanghai free trade zone.

Second, the local health authority would have to take the private sector into account when making its local health resource planning. At least 20% of the quota must be set aside for the private sector in terms of hospital equipment and other indexes.

In October 2014, a government guideline for private insurance was released.[33] More insurance products would be developed to meet the demand for better financial coverage of health care. Medical liability insurance, sometimes known as medical malpractice insurance, will be developed. These insurance schemes can be very helpful in settling

---

[30] Yan Xiaolin, et al., "Commercial Health Insurance under the New Healthcare Reform".
[31] <http://news.xinhuanet.com/politics/2013-11/15/c_118164235.htm> (accessed 26 February 2015).
[32] <http://www.nhfpc.gov.cn/tigs/s7846/201401/239ae12d249c4e38a5e2de45 7ee20253.shtml> (accessed 26 February 2015).
[33] <http://www.gov.cn/zhengce/content/2014-11/17/content_9210.htm> (accessed 26 February 2015).

medical malpractice disputes. The National Health and Family Planning Commission has plans for 100% coverage of medical liability insurance for tertiary public hospitals in the near future. It was reported in March 2016 that the 100% coverage for tertiary public hospitals had been achieved and 100% of public hospitals will be covered by 2020.[34]

In this document, private insurers are encouraged to manage social health insurance and other complementary social health insurance. Local governments may buy services from private health insurers to manage their social insurance commitments. Public hospitals are encouraged to appoint providers of private health insurance.

In January 2015, the State Council endorsed the guideline for health resource planning for the 2015–2020 period.[35] The establishment of private hospitals and hospitals with mixed ownership is encouraged.

Another policy guideline for regulating the practices of doctors was released by the National Health and Family Planning Commission in January 2015.[36] This policy is to encourage the mobility of doctors and the entry of the private sector, which is short of human resources to provide health-care services.

Recent Developments of the Private Sector in the Chinese Health-care System

The entry of the private sector in the Chinese health-care system took two forms. One is the privatisation of hospitals. China Resource Healthcare Company has started to build a hospital chain since 2011. By the end of 2014, there were at least six hospitals and over 7,000

---

[34] <http://china.caixin.com/2016-03-28/100925607.html> (accessed 24 July 2016).
[35] <http://finance.sina.com.cn/chanjing/cyxw/20150120/011921334930.shtml> (accessed 26 February 2015).
[36] <http://www.nhfpc.gov.cn/yzygj/s3577/201501/8663861edc7d40db91810ebf0ab 996df.shtml> (accessed 29 May 2015).

hospital beds in five provinces under China Resource Healthcare.[37] Most of these hospitals were once public hospitals.[38]

Pharmaceutical companies are also among the first group of buyers for hospitals. Foshun Pharma has also attempted to establish a hospital chain; it now has over 2,000 beds. Most hospitals under Foshun Pharma were previously private hospitals.[39]

Another is public-private partnership. One outstanding recent example is the "mixed ownership" pilot in public hospital reform. "Mixed ownership" refers to institutional investors from either public or private sectors in public enterprises including public hospitals. The arrangement is believed to be a win-win solution for both public and private sectors given that public hospitals have the advantage of human resources (that is, more qualified doctors and nurses), while the private sector has larger financial capacities to invest in public hospitals. Some insurance companies have started to buy out hospitals. For example, Sunshine Insurance Group has bought 51% of shares of the biggest public hospital in Weifang city in Shandong, one of the public hospital reform pilots.[40]

Hospitals with mixed ownership are also subject to less regulation in the local health resource plan compared to that of private hospitals.[41] In April 2014, a public hospital in Hunan province had been selected as a pilot for mixed ownership reform.[42] While the government has a

---

[37] <http://www.yicai.com/news/2014/12/4057651.html> (accessed 26 February 2015).

[38] <http://finance.ifeng.com/a/20140710/12689324_0.shtml> (accessed 26 February 2015).

[39] <http://www.cn-healthcare.com/article/20140818/content-459545-all.html> (accessed 25 February 2015).

[40] *China Times*, 14 May 2016, <http://www.chinatimes.cc/article/56735.html> (accessed 28 May 2015).

[41] <http://jingji.21cbh.com/2014/3-12/0MMDA2NTFfMTA5MzE0Mg.html> (accessed 2 March 2015).

[42] <http://news.xinhuanet.com/local/2014-04/17/c_1110290117.htm> (accessed 26 May 2016).

Table 7-2:   Cases of Mixed Ownership in Public Hospitals in 2014

Hospital Name	Province	External Investors (from Private Sector)	External Investors' Share of Ownership
Peking University International Hospital	Beijing	Founder Group	85%
Sixth Xiangya Hospital of Central South University	Hunan	Meixihu Group	80%
Taizhou Zanyang Hospital	Zhejiang	Fosun Group	75%
Sixth Subsidiary Sun Yat-sen University Hospital	Guangdong	GL Capital Group	60%
Xuzhou No. 3 People's Hospital	Jiangsu	Sanpower Group	80%
Yangguang Ronghe Hospital	Shandong	Sunshine Insurance Group	51%

Source: Compiled by the author from various news reports.

51% shareholding of this hospital, private investors hold the rest of the shares.

Table 7-2 lists other cases of mixed ownership in public hospitals in 2014. In all these cases, private investors hold more than 50% of the shares, with the rest owned by the government, universities or other public hospitals.

Some local pilots have started to allow doctors to practise in more than one hospital. In Beijing, doctors have been able to practise in a second hospital without the endorsement of their registered hospital since 2014. In 2014, over 1,100 doctors were practising in more than one hospital in Beijing, four times the number in 2013.[43]

Other forms of public-private partnership are the operate-transfer model. For example, by the end of 2015, Phoenix Healthcare Group, the largest privately owned hospital group, manages about 60 health-care providers including three tertiary hospitals. Phoenix Healthcare Group

---

[43] <http://epaper.nandu.com/epaper/A/html/2015-01/12/content_3374299.htm?div=0> (accessed 24 February 2015).

also had over 5,700 beds by 2015.[44] Many of these hospitals are still publicly owned but they are managed by the Phoenix Healthcare Group. In this mode, the input from the private sector is to improve the management of infrastructure, procurement and personnel management.

For private insurance, private insurers are allowed to work with social health insurers to improve affordability of health care. In August 2012, a government guideline on the "catastrophic medical insurance programme" ("*Dabing Yibao*") was released.[45] The catastrophic medical insurance programme is a supplementary insurance programme to extend the coverage of insurance by increasing both the rate and the upper limit of reimbursement.

In this guideline, social insurers are advised to reinsure with private insurance companies to improve the coverage while the government will take the lead role in designing and managing the "catastrophic medical insurance programme". In 2014, the "catastrophic medical insurance programme" covered about 400 million people in 28 provinces.[46]

The initiation of the catastrophic medical insurance programme was motivated by first, the need to improve the affordability of health-care services. The programme, which focuses on relieving patients burdened by catastrophic medical expenditure, will improve the depth of the insurance coverage by increasing both the reimbursement rate and the upper limit of the reimbursement.

Second is the complementarity of private insurers and social health insurers.[47] While social insurers have huge financial resources, with

---

[44] *Caixin Weekly*, 24 May 2016, <http://weekly.caixin.com/2016-05-20/100945675.html> (accessed 28 May 2016).

[45] <http://www.mof.gov.cn/zhengwuxinxi/zhengcefabu/201208/t20120831_679663.htm> (accessed 24 May 2016).

[46] <http://companies.caixin.com/2014-07-09/100701481.html> (accessed 24 May 2016).

[47] Sun Zhigang, "The Catastrophic Medical Insurance as the Key Point of Improving Affordability of Health Care", <http://theory.people.com.cn/n/2013/0125/c40531-20326536.html> (accessed 24 July 2016). Note: Sun was the director of the health reform office in the State Council in 2013.

accumulated surpluses of BHI reaching over RMB918 billion in 2014, compared to RMB127 billion in 2005,[48] private insurers have the professional expertise to work out the financial risks of health insurance policies for catastrophic health-care spending.

Discussions

While some of the constraints for the development of the private sector have been removed in the recent policy initiatives, institutional constraints pertaining to the development of the private sector in the Chinese health-care system remain.

Policy implementation for the deregulation is still an issue. The private sector is still restricted by regulations in the health service market. The regulatory framework is still in favour of public hospitals. For example, apart from Beijing and Zhejiang provinces, in most localities, the regulation on doctors' dual practice has yet to be reformed.[49]

There are still institutional constraints for the development of private insurers and private hospitals. For example, the government still imposes strict regulation over private insurers' policies for the newly initiated catastrophic medical insurance programme. Private insurers do not have much say in insurance policy design and are usually paid by commission for managing the fund. The commission paid to private insurers is a proportion of the premium paid to social health insurance.

For instance, in Xiamen city, private insurers are paid at the maximum 3% of the premium. The government will subsidise private insurers to keep the budget balanced should there be any financial losses to the scheme.[50] In some cities such as Hangzhou, it is the local

[48] *China Human Resources and Social Security Yearbook*, various years and budget report 2014, Ministry of Finance.

[49] <http://epaper.nandu.com/epaper/A/html/2015-01/12/content_3374299.htm?div=0> (accessed 24 February 2015).

[50] Qiu Yunlin and Huang Guowu, "The Mechanism for the Catastrophic Medical Insurance Program: International and China experiences", *Zhongzhou xuekan*, vol. 1, 2014, pp. 61–66.

social insurer and not the private insurer who is involved in/manages the catastrophic medical insurance programme.[51]

Unlike countries such as Australia, Singapore and the United States, there are no tax rebates for consumers who buy private health insurance in China. Private insurance can play a bigger role if tax rebate policy is available.[52]

For the hospital sector, the progress in public hospital ownership reform has reportedly been slowing down since local governments have concerns about possible loss of state-owned assets.[53]

It remains a question whether affordability will be improved after the entry of the private sector in the health-care service market.[54] Given the nature of the health-care service, consumers have not enough knowledge or information to judge the quality of the service. Some experts are therefore concerned that profit-driven service providers and entrance of private investment could work in the reverse and "result in the escalation of health-care cost, inefficient use of pharmaceutical and high-tech diagnostic tests…".[55]

In principle, competition among service providers can increase the bargaining power of the "purchaser" (i.e. health insurers) who controls the health expenditure. However, the perverse incentives and low capacity of social health insurers in China are issues to be addressed for

---

[51] Qiu Yunlin and Huang Guowu, "The Mechanism for the Catastrophic Medical Insurance Program".

[52] A number of big cities have been selected as pilot for tax rebate for private health insurance since January 2016, <http://szs.mof.gov.cn/zhengwuxinxi/zhengce-fabu/201512/t20151211_1609629.html> (accessed 24 July 2016).

[53] Caixin Weekly, 23 May 2016. <http://weekly.caixin.com/2016-05-20/100945675.html> (accessed 28 May 2016).

[54] For some detailed policy suggestions, see Åke Blomqvist and Qian Jiwei, "China's Future Health Care system: What role for private production and financing?" International Journal of Healthcare Technology and Management, forthcoming.

[55] Winnie Yip and William Hsiao, "Harnessing the Privatization of China's Fragmented Health-care Delivery".

the policymakers.[56] The entry of private insurance can be one reform option to improve the capacity of and set the right incentives for health insurers.

---

[56] See the discussion on social health insurance in Chapter 5 of this book. See also a general discussion in Ramesh M, Wu Xun and Alex He Jingwei, "Health Governance and Health Care Reforms in China".

Chapter 8

Regulating Tobacco Uses

Regulating Tobacco Use[1]

Tobacco use is one of the most significant public health issues in China, a policy area that needs an efficient regulatory system. Smoking is recognised as one of the major causes of lung cancer, stroke and heart disease. The number of deaths caused by tobacco use in China is currently 1.2 million a year.[2] There are 350 million smokers in China, among which 52.9% of males and 2.4% of females over 15 years old are regular smokers.[3] The treatment costs for acute myocardial infarction and stroke caused by tobacco use in 2012 was estimated to be US$8 billion in health-care costs; it is said to lead to reduced productivity, premature death and others.[4] The total economic costs of adverse health effects of tobacco usage in China were estimated

---

[1]This chapter draws materials from Qian Jiwei, "Tobacco Control in China: Institutions, bureaucratic noncompliance and policy ineffectiveness", in Kjeld Erik Brøsdgaard (ed.), *Chinese Politics as Fragmented Authoritarianism*, London, Routledge, 2016, pp. 56–76.
[2]Li Cheng, *The Political Mapping of China's Tobacco Industry and Anti-Smoking Campaign*, Washington, Brookings Institution, John L Thornton China Centre Monograph Series, 2012.
[3]Qian Jiwei, "Tobacco Control in China".
[4]Yang Gonghuan, et al., "The Road to Effective Tobacco Control in China", *The Lancet*, vol. 385, Issue 9972, 2015, pp. 1019–1028.

at about US$28.9 billion in 2008 and have been increasing ever since.[5] These costs include health expenditure for treating smoke related diseases and costs that are associated with premature death. There are also about 740 million people who are regularly exposed to second hand smoke.[6] Notably, China was also the world's biggest producer of cigarettes, accounting for 44% of total world consumption in 2014.[7] In 2020, the number of deaths caused by smoking is expected to hit two million in China.[8]

In recent years, China has started a number of regulatory initiatives at both the central and local levels. While some achievements have been made, the implementation is not very effective in general. The low capacity of regulatory agencies for tobacco control is one important reason for the ineffectiveness of policy implementation. Incentives of regulators and the institutional arrangement for implementing tobacco control policies could throw light on the ineffectiveness of policy enforcement.

International experiences of tobacco control

Tobacco use is one of the most preventable causes of death. International experiences of government intervention/government regulation have been proven to be very effective for tobacco control.[9] Governments can intervene from either the demand side or the supply side of tobacco use through regulation, legislation or economic intervention. Supply-side policies include reducing subsidies for tobacco

---

[5] Yang Lian, et al., "Economic Costs Attributable to Smoking in China: Update and an 8-year comparison 2000–2008", *Tobacco Control*, vol. 20, 2011, pp. 266–72.

[6] Yang Gonghuan and Hu Angang, *Tobacco Control and China's Future (Kongyan yu zhongguo weilai)*, (in Chinese), Beijing, Economic Daily Press, 2011.

[7] *China Youth Daily*, 26 November 2015, <http://www.chinanews.com/gn/2015/11-26/7641921.shtml> (accessed 22 May 2016).

[8] Anita Lee and Jiang Yuan, "Tobacco Control Programs in China", in Hu Teh-wei (ed.) *Tobacco Control Policy Analysis in China*, Singapore, World Scientific, 2008, pp. 33–56.

[9] World Health Organisation, *Building Blocks for Tobacco Control, A Handbook*, Geneva, World Health Organisation, 2004.

leaf production, suppressing the illegal trade of tobacco products and providing support for economically viable alternative activities.

On the demand side, government policies in general can be divided into three groups: policies on price, image and exposure.[10] The first set of policies increases cigarette and tobacco prices through raising taxes. Increasing cigarette price is also known to be more effective in relation to teenagers and the poor since they are more price-sensitive.[11] There is also evidence that people in low-income countries are more sensitive to cigarette price increases than people in high-income countries.[12] The second includes the enforcement of regulations regarding the display of health warning labels on cigarette packages.[13] The third refers to policies on exposure, which includes banning smoking in public spaces and banning cigarette advertisements in mass media. Comprehensive bans on all advertising and promotion have proven to be effective.[14]

The Rise of the Regulatory State and Tobacco Control in China

To borrow an economic term, tobacco users have very large negative "externalities". The social costs of their behaviour are much larger than the private costs imposed on themselves as many people suffer from second hand smoke. In this case, government intervention is believed to be most effective in the arena of tobacco control.

The Chinese government has been regulating tobacco use for a long time now. It influences the price of tobacco by imposing taxes on tobacco leaf, cigarette production, consumption and distribution. The Chinese government influences price by imposing taxes on tobacco leaf, cigarette production, consumption and distribution. Tobacco

---

[10] World Health Organisation. *Building Blocks for Tobacco Control, A Handbook*.

[11] WHO, MPOWER brochures — Raise taxes on tobacco.

[12] WHO, MPOWER brochures — Raise taxes on tobacco.

[13] World Health Organisation, *WHO Report on the Global Tobacco Epidemic*, Geneva, World Health Organisation, 2009.

[14] World Health Organisation, *Building Blocks for Tobacco Control, A Handbook*.

leaf producers are subject to a 20% tobacco leaf tax and the tax revenue generated is allocated to the local government. For distributors, a consumption tax is set at either 36% or 56%, depending on the producer's price range. Wholesalers are subject to an 11% tax, while quantity-based consumption tax is set at RMB0.16 per pack.[15] Cigarette producers need to pay a 17% value-added tax. Apart from tobacco leaf tax and value-added tax, other taxes are fully under the control of the central government as part of its revenue. Beyond taxes, wholesale price mark-up ranging from 15% to 34% is imposed at the wholesale level, depending on the range of producer prices.

At the national level, regulations and laws have been enacted to control tobacco use. A landmark tobacco control legislation — Law of the People's Republic of China on Tobacco Monopoly — was passed in 1991. Under this law, cigarette advertisements in China are banned in national and international TV and radio programmes, newspapers and magazines. Smoking is also banned in selected public transport and public places. In 2005, China ratified the World Health Organisation's Framework Convention on Tobacco Control (FCTC) initiated by the World Health Organisation (WHO). The FCTC now has 180 member countries.[16]

Local tobacco control regulations have recently been implemented in some big cities. For example, in Hangzhou, smoking has been banned in most public spaces since March 2010. The Shanghai government has similarly banned smoking in almost all public spaces such as schools and hospitals since March 2010 in anticipation of the Shanghai Expo. Smoking is also banned in public spaces in Guangzhou since September 2010 before the 2010 Asian Games. Since 2008, at least 12 cities have enacted or amended subnational smoke-free public

---

[15] On 8 May 2015, a new set of tobacco tax policy was announced. The tax rate for wholesalers has been increased from 5% to 11%. Quantity-based consumption tax has also been adjusted to RMB0.16 per pack from RMB0.06 per pack (20 cigarettes per pack).

[16] BBC Chinese, 1 June 2015, <http://www.bbc.com/zhongwen/simp/world/2015/06/150601_anti_smoking_measures> (accessed 22 May 2016).

places legislations or regulations. In June 2015, Beijing's smoke-free regulations, the country's strictest tobacco control law, took effect, leaving all indoor and many outdoor public spaces in Beijing 100% smoke-free.[17] Eighteen cities had banned smoking in public places by the end of 2015.[18]

The Effectiveness of Regulation Enforcement

The enforcement of laws and regulations for tobacco control however has not been very effective. At the national level, China has been relatively slow in implementing its obligations under the FCTC to amend existing laws and regulations to limit the extent of exposure of smoking in at least two areas: banning of all smoking activities in all public spaces and specifying the penalties for violating tobacco control regulations or laws. In addition to controlling exposure, current laws have to be amended to implement the relevant standards for the inclusion of warning labels on cigarette packages and to ban all advertising, promotion and sponsorship of the tobacco industry in all media.

As of December 2016, a national smoke-free law that satisfies FCTC requirements had yet to be approved. The draft, which was in the process of deliberation, has not satisfied the requirements of the FCTC. For example, smoking is allowed in restricted areas in many public spaces such as restaurants and teahouses according to this draft.[19]

The Chinese Centre for Disease Control and Prevention (CDC) has also reported that the effectiveness of current tobacco control policies is unsatisfactory, with a score of only 37 out of 100 points for the implementation of the six major policies in the WHO MPOWER

---

[17] World Health Organisation. *Smoke-free Policies in China*, Geneva, World Health Organisation, 2015.
[18] *Workers' Daily*, 1 May 2016, <http://news.163.com/16/0501/07/BLVCSCKK 00014AEE.html> (accessed 22 May 2016).
[19] *Beijing News*, 3 May 2016, <http://news.xinhuanet.com/health/2016-05/03/c_ 128951405.htm> (accessed 22 May 2016).

package.[20] MPOWER is an abbreviation of six policy guidelines: monitoring tobacco use and prevention policies; protecting people from tobacco smoke; offering help to quit tobacco use; warning about the dangers of tobacco; enforcing bans on tobacco advertising, promotion and sponsorship; and raising taxes on tobacco.[21]

According to the Global Adult Tobacco Survey conducted by the WHO in conjunction with the Chinese CDC and US Centre for Diseases Control and Prevention in China, the adult smoking rate and exposure rate to second hand smoke in 2010 almost equalled the rate in 2002, suggesting that the enforcement of the newly initiated tobacco control regulations in this period was not very effective. In addition, according to this survey, over 60% of smokers continued to smoke despite the warning labels on cigarette packs.[22]

Only one fourth of adults in China were aware of the health hazards of tobacco use and only 16% of current smokers planned to or were thinking about quitting in the next 12 months.[23] The progress of tobacco control legislation at the local level that complies with FCTC requirements has also been very limited. One outstanding example is the failure of the Nanchang People's Congress to pass tobacco control legislation twice in 2010. As of January 2016, a third draft of the legislation was still being reviewed.[24] Furthermore, except for Beijing's 2015 regulation, most local regulations fail to meet FCTC requirements. For example, FCTC Article 8 requires "universal protection from tobacco smoking in all indoor public places, indoor workplaces and public transport". However, in Shanghai's tobacco control regulations,

---

[20]Yang Gonghuan and Hu Angang, *Tobacco Control and China's Future*.
[21]See WHO website <http://www.who.int/tobacco/mpower/en/> (accessed 22 May 2016).
[22]Chinese Centre for Disease Control and Prevention, *Global Adult Tobacco Survey China Country Report*, Beijing, Chinese Centre for Disease Control and Prevention, 2011.
[23]Chinese Centre for Disease Control and Prevention, *Global Adult Tobacco Survey China Country Report*.
[24]JiangNan Dushi Bao, "Quanguo 14 Cheng, Nanchang Shinei Xiyanlu zuigao" (Nanchang has the highest smoking rate among 14 cities in China), 8 January 2016.

for example, selective public places are set to be smoke-free and smoking is allowed to some degree in the remaining public places, including restaurants, bars and offices.[25]

The enforcement of tobacco control regulations at the local level has also been ineffective. For example, between 1998 and 2013 in Shenzhen, not one single person was fined for violating tobacco control regulations.[26] Similarly, no one had been fined for a period of 10 months in Guangzhou for violating tobacco control law after it was enacted in 2010.[27]

Coordination in the enforcement of tobacco regulations is another important issue that needs to be resolved. At the central level, a group consisting of eight government departments, "the leading small group for the Implementation Coordination Mechanism of FCTC", was initiated by the State Council in April 2007 to coordinate the implementation of FCTC policies.[28] This small leading group announced a plan for tobacco control between 2012 and 2015. However, the plan has failed to achieve some of its key targets, such as reducing the number of smokers and the volume of cigarette consumption.[29]

At the local level, there are usually more than a dozen government departments involved in the enforcement of tobacco control regulations and coordination is a problem. For example, in Shenzhen and Guangzhou, there are 12 and 15 government departments, respectively, involved in regulation enforcement. They include the bureaus in charge

---

[25] Qian Jiwei, *Tobacco Control in China: Institutions, bureaucratic noncompliance and policy ineffectiveness.*

[26] *Yangcheng Evening News*, "Shenzhen kongyan tiaoli chutai shinian weichuju yizhang fadan" (Shenzhen government has not issued a single fine after releasing tobacco control regulation for 10 years), 27 December 2013.

[27] *Yangcheng Evening News*, "Kongyan tiaoli Shishi 10 geyue Guangzou kaichu shouzhang fadan" (Guangzhou government has issued the first fine after releasing tobacco control regulation for 10 months), 1 July 2011.

[28] Qian Jiwei, *Tobacco Control in China: Institutions, bureaucratic noncompliance and policy ineffectiveness.*

[29] *People's Daily*, "Woguo Shouge Kongyan Guihua Wei dabiao" (China has missed the first tobacco control target), 27 January 2016.

of health, education, transportation, public security, city urban administration, market supervision, industry and commerce, among others.

Similarly, the cigarette tax has had little effect on reducing cigarette consumption. Currently, the cigarette tax in China was about 56% of retail price in 2015,[30] while it was 63% in Thailand and 69% in Singapore.[31] Internationally, average cigarette tax at the retail level is about 65%, while it is much higher in OECD countries. For the most purchased cigarette brand in China, the tax rate per pack is about 36%, which is significantly lower than the international standard of about 50–60%[32] and certainly much lower than the 76% tax in Singapore.

Why Tobacco Control Regulations Are Not Effective in China: Capacity and Incentives

There are two major reasons for the ineffectiveness of tobacco control regulation enforcement. First, the capacity of the regulatory agencies is inadequate. The fund for the National Office of Tobacco Control (NOTC) for surveillance and monitoring of tobacco was about RMB10 million or an annual RMB0.01 per capita in recent years, much less than that in other countries.[33] For example, in the United States, the budget for surveillance and monitoring of tobacco was $0.2 per capita, or $60 million.[34] The human resources for tobacco control in China are also pathetic. There are only four permanent professional staff and 16 contract staff under NOTC in 2007, four years after establishment.[35] In 2009, NOTC had only 27 staff.[36] At the local level,

---

[30] <http://china.caixin.com/2015-06-01/100815082.html> (accessed 8 October 2016).

[31] World Health Organisation, *WHO report on the Global Tobacco Epidemic.*

[32] World Health Organisation, *WHO report on the Global Tobacco Epidemic.*

[33] <http://news.xinhuanet.com/finance/2015-11-26/c_128471320.htm> (accessed 25 July 2016).

[34] <http://www.cdc.gov/mmwr/preview/mmwrhtml/mm6424a5.htm> (accessed 22 May 2016).

[35] Anita Lee and Jiang Yuan, "Tobacco Control Programs in China".

[36] Yang Gonghuan and Hu Angang, *Tobacco Control and China's Future.*

the shortage of resources is also a serious issue. For example, there were only five invigilators in Guangzhou for the enforcement of tobacco control regulations in 2015.[37]

Second, the ineffectiveness of tobacco control regulations can be explained by the incentives of bureaucrats, as bureaucrats not only set the regulations, but also implement them. Compared to bureaucrats in Mao's era, bureaucrats have become even more influential and have the incentives to pursue their goals strategically in the process of policy implementation.

Institutional arrangement for regulating tobacco uses

The incentives of bureaucrats are configured by two institutions: the performance evaluation system for government officials and the government monopoly over the tobacco industry.[38]

The first institution is the performance evaluation system for local government officials, a reason for local government officials' weak incentives to enforce regulations. Performance evaluation system can be considered as an institutional response to the fragmented structure of government departments since officials are accountable for selected performance indexes under this system.

Appointment, promotion and demotion of local bureaucrats are decided according to whether they have fulfilled what is required of them in their job performance. Local officials in China are likely to be promoted based on GDP growth rate and fiscal revenue.[39] Local government has a strong incentive to allocate fiscal resources to build local

---

[37] *China Youth Daily*, 26 November 2015, <http://www.chinanews.com/gn/2015/11-26/7641921.shtml> (accessed 22 May 2016).

[38] Qian Jiwei, *Tobacco Control in China: Institutions, bureaucratic noncompliance and policy ineffectiveness.*

[39] See Li Hongbin and Zhou Li-An, "Political Turnover and Economic Performance: The incentive role of personnel control in China", *Journal of Public Economics*, vol. 89, Issue 9–10, 2005, pp. 1743–1762 and Victor Shih, et al., "Getting Ahead in the Communist Party: Explaining the advancement of Central Committee members in China", *American Political Science Review*, vol. 106, no. 1, 2012, pp. 166–187.

infrastructure in order to promote economic growth and broaden tax bases.

However, the fiscal capacity of many local governments is not large enough to cover their expenditure. In recent years, local governments are responsible for over 80% of government expenditure, while they are only assigned with about 50% of government revenue. Figure 8-1 shows this mismatch between revenue assignment and expenditure responsibility.

For many local governments, the fiscal revenue from the tobacco industry is extremely important and the enforcement of tobacco control regulations may affect their local fiscal revenue. For example, tax revenue together with profit from the tobacco sector amounted to 58% of total fiscal revenue in Yunnan province in 2010.[40] In Hunan and Guizhou provinces, the tobacco industry contributed 29% and 23%

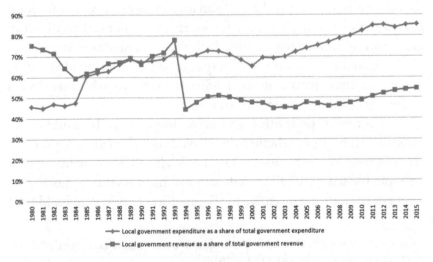

Figure 8-1:   Local Government's Share in Fiscal Revenue and Expenditure

Source: Ministry of Finance, budget report, various years.

---

[40] STMA, "Guojia shuishou zhong yancaoye de qingkuang" (Tobacco industry role in government tax revenue), 2011, <http://www.tobacco.gov.cn/html/21/2106/210603/21060301/3758615_n.html> (accessed 24 November 2015).

of total fiscal revenue in 2006, respectively.[41] After the repealing of the agriculture tax in 2006, the tobacco leaf tax has been especially important for local public finance of counties in the rural areas. Currently, 24 of the 31 provinces in China grow tobacco leaves. Tobacco leaf tax is a significant source of fiscal revenue for 185 out of 510 national level poverty-stricken counties.[42]

In some provinces, tobacco leaf tax may not be a very significant part of fiscal revenue, but other types of taxes from the tobacco industry, such as value-added taxes, account for an important share of local government revenue. For example, in Jiangxi province, taxes from the tobacco industry, including value-added tax and corporate income tax, contribute about 40% of total tax revenue from the manufacturing sector in 2010.[43] Even for the economically developed regions, the share of tax contributed by the tobacco industry in government revenue is also large when compared to other industries. For example, the tobacco industry, as the largest contributor in the manufacturing sector, accounted for over one-third of total tax revenue from all industries in Shanghai in 2011.[44]

As the tobacco industry plays an important role in the local economy, local officials who have incentives to maximise fiscal revenue, may not be willing to fully enforce tobacco control policies. In 2015, the tobacco industry contributed RMB1.09 trillion to the Chinese government, accounting for about 7.16% of total fiscal revenue.[45]

The second institution configuring bureaucrats' incentives is the government's monopoly of the tobacco industry. This is in particular the case at the central level. The State Tobacco Monopoly Administration

---

[41] *Beijing Review*, "Yancaoye, bei kongzhi de juren" (Tobacco industry, a giant under control), 28 January 2010.

[42] Hu Teh-wei, et al., "The Role of Taxation in Tobacco Control and its Potential Economic Impact in China", *Tobacco Control*, vol. 19, no. 1, 2010, pp. 58–64.

[43] *Jiangxi Statistical Yearbook*, Jiangxi, Yichun, China Statistics Press, 2011.

[44] *Shanghai Statistical Yearbook*, Shanghai, Shanghai People's Publishing House, 2012.

[45] *Economic Daily*, "Yancaoye Shangjiao Caizhen Chao Wanyiyuan" (Tobacco industry has submitted over 1 trillion as profits and taxes), 18 January 2016.

(STMA) is both a government department and state-owned monopoly of the tobacco industry in China. Known as China National Tobacco Corporation (CNTC),[46] STMA has secured a place in the leading small group for implementing FCTC obligations. In 2008, MIIT, whose deputy minister is also the head of STMA, replaced the NDRC as the coordinator for implementing FCTC obligations (Table 8-1). Steered by a deputy minister, MIIT is responsible for the day-to-day compliance of FCTC requirements.[47] STMA also participates in the drafting of national guidelines and legislation for tobacco control.

With the MIIT playing the role of the coordinator of the small leading group, the incentive to enforce the FCTC can be expected to be low since the regulators of the tobacco industry represent the interests of the regulated (i.e. 'regulatory capture'[48]).

Discussions

Regulatory agents at both local and central levels have been inefficient in implementing tobacco control policies. From earlier discussions, the development of the regulatory regime for tobacco control has been constrained by both the capacity, such as the shortage of financial and human resources, and the incentive structure of the regulators which is subject to the performance evaluation system. At the central level, "regulatory capture" occurs in the process of implementing tobacco control policies.

To improve the effectiveness of tobacco control regulation enforcement, the performance evaluation system for government officials must be reformed to make them accountable for the outcomes of tobacco control policies and an independent agency responsible for tobacco control would be needed to address the "regulatory capture" issue.

---

[46] See <http://www.tobacco.gov.cn/html/> (accessed 25 July 2016).
[47] Matthew Kohrman, "New Steps for Tobacco Control in and Outside China", *Asia-Pacific Journal of Public Health*, vol. 22, 2010, pp. 189–96.
[48] George Stigler, "The Theory of Economic Regulation".

Table 8-1: Division of Labour Among Eight Ministries in the Leading Small Group for Implementing FCTC in China

Ministry	Division of Responsibilities
Ministry of Industry and Information Technology	Implement the work plan, research the transition of and the alternatives to the tobacco industry, and report on performance and exchange information.
Ministry of Health (CDC, NOTC)	Protect the public from exposure to smoking, promote public education, monitor prevalence levels of tobacco use and communicate with the FCTC Secretariat.
Ministry of Foreign Affairs	Advise other agencies on China's obligations under the treaty, lead PRC's official delegations to FCTC conferences, coordinate Hong Kong and Macao Special Administrative Regions' compliance with the treaty and promote foreign exchange and cooperation.
Ministry of Finance	Develop strategies to reduce the demand for tobacco, establish price and tax measures, and research financial resources and assistance mechanisms.
STMA (CNTC)	Regulate the packaging and label of tobacco products (printing warning labels on cigarette packs), disclose tobacco production information, ensure higher taxation on tobacco products, combat illicit trade in tobacco and regulate tobacco advertising.
State Administration for Industry and Commerce	Regulate tobacco advertising and combat illicit tobacco trade.
General Administration of Customs	Combat illicit trade in tobacco products (mainly smuggling).
General Administration of Quality Supervision, Inspection and Quarantine	Package and label tobacco products.

Source: Compiled from Li Cheng, *The Political Mapping of China's Tobacco Industry and Anti-Smoking Campaign*.

Chapter 9

Conclusions and Discussions

From the discussions in this book, a regulatory state is evidently emerging in the Chinese health-care system with the initiation and implementation of a number of regulations; regulatory agencies have been vested with more authority and new regulatory agencies established. In some policy areas, some measurable indexes have been employed for enforcing regulations. For example, financial surpluses of social insurance funds are subject to certain measurable indexes (e.g. balanced and accumulated surpluses, in principle, should amount to at least half-a-year reimbursement). Another example of using indexes is related to the competition policy where market concentration ratio is used as an important index for policy enforcement. Prices for patent drugs are also considered as an important index under AML and overpricing may be seen as an evidence of abusing market dominance.

However, as shown in this book, while there are many regulations in place, in most policy areas, the low policy enforcement capacity of the regulatory agencies is a major constraint. One obvious area is the lack of human resources for the regulatory agencies in the pharmaceutical sector and public health. Low capacity could be a result of low financial input. Health expenditure and government health expenditure in China accounted for about 6% and 1.9% of GDP in 2015 respectively. These numbers are significantly below OECD average. For example, health expenditure and government health expenditure as a share of GDP on average in OECD countries were a respective 8.9% and 6.5% in 2012.[1] With growing economic size and income level, the capacity constraint of regulating the Chinese health-care system will be alleviated to some degree with more human and fiscal resources allocated to the Chinese health sector.

This book also shows that the incentives of regulators may not be fully compatible with public interest. For example, regulatory agencies may not want to enforce tobacco control policies as the industry contributes to a significant part of local fiscal revenue.

The more important question however is the institutional constraints for regulatory agencies. In the words of famous economist Dani Rodrik, institutional arrangements for the regulatory agents are likely to be the "binding constraint".[2] At the horizontal level, institutional arrangements are likely to be fragmented among many government departments. At the vertical level, incentives for the local enforcers are not aligned with the objectives of regulatory agencies at the central level. These institutional and incentive constraints are not limited to the health-care system. A similar situation prevails for environmental policy enforcement and tax administration enforcement in China. For example, research has shown that the performance evaluation system has adverse effects on environmental policy enforcement.[3] Likewise, in the policy area of tax administration, decentralisation of tax administration is the major reason for the development of a rule-based tax system in China.[4]

---

[1] OECD health statistics.

[2] Dani Rodrik, *One Economics, Many Recipes: Globalization, institutions, and economic growth*, Princeton, Princeton University Press, 2008.

[3] See Zhou Xueguang, et al., "A Behavioral Model of 'Muddling Through' in the Chinese Bureaucracy: The case of environmental protection", *The China Journal*, vol. 70, no. 1, 2013, pp. 120–147; Wu Jing, et al., "Incentives and Outcomes: China's environmental policy", *NBER working paper*, no. 18754, 2013.

[4] See Cui Wei, "Administrative Decentralization and Tax Compliance: A transactional cost perspective", *University of Toronto Law Journal*, vol. 65, no. 3, 2015, pp. 186–238.

A Closer Look at the Institutional Arrangements of the Regulators

From the literature of organisational economics, in principle, the information structure and degree of conflicts in tasks within an organisation determine the optimal allocation of authority.[5] As long as the incentives conflict between the principal and agents is not too substantial, agents with better access to information would be granted the authority. In this case, authority allocation is a policy instrument for the principal to take advantage of local knowledge/information. In addition, when there are multiple tasks to be fulfilled, the authority to deal with interest-conflicting tasks should be delegated to different agencies. This is to avoid conflict of interest and improve accountability since it is easier to measure agencies' performance with focused missions.

How to reform institutional arrangements for regulating the health-care system can be understood from the perspective of allocating decision-making right in organisations.[6] The decision-making right in regulation can be allocated between central and local governments, or among different government departments at a given level of government. Treating government departments and different levels

---

[5] Patrick Bolton and Mathias Dewatripont, "Authority in Organizations: A survey" and Robert Gibbons, Niko Matouschek and John Roberts, "Decisions in Organizations", in Robert Gibbons and John Roberts (eds.), *Handbook of The Handbook of Organizational Economics*, Princeton, Princeton University Press, 2012.

[6] See Jean Tirole, "The Internal Organization of Government", *Oxford Economic Papers*, 1994, pp. 1–29; Philippe Aghion and Jean Tirole, "Formal and Real Authority in Organizations", *Journal of Political Economy*, 1997, pp. 1–29. For a similar discussion of Chinese social policies, see Qian Jiwei, "Reforming with 'Separation of Authority' in the China's Social Welfare System", Working paper, 2016. For an analysis in the context of the Chinese health-care system, see Qian Jiwei, "Reallocating Authority in the Chinese Health System: An institutional perspective", *Journal of Asian Public Policy*, vol. 8, no. 1, 2015, pp. 19–35.

of governments as self-interested players is also consistent with the literature on public choice.[7]

Information in the regulatory system can be considered in two dimensions. First is the degree to which local knowledge or local adaption is relevant to policy enforcement. Second is the degree to which policy enforcement relies on professional expertise.

Vertically, the allocation of decision-making right is contingent on the trade-off between information and interests. Local government may have its own agenda, which is not always consistent with the policymaker's incentives at the central level, even with the performance evaluation system.

In some policy areas, local governments may have better access to local information/local knowledge. In other policy areas, centralising the authority of decision making in policy design and policy implementation may have large gains from synergies (i.e. economics of scale/scope)[8] or a better capacity to solicit the expertise of professionals.

Horizontally, the considerations for the allocation of decision-making right is similar. The trade-off between interest and information is critical and institutions such as joint ministerial conferences or small leading groups may need to take into account the structure of information and interests of all stakeholders.

From the perspective of conflicting interests among different agents, some government departments are more likely to be "captured" by the interest of the regulated, which is not compatible with the regulator's objective. From the information dimension, some government departments have better access to information/local knowledge or have better professional expertise. They are in a better position to make decisions in the implementation of the regulation.

---

[7] For example, see Dennis Mueller, *Public Choice III*, Cambridge, Cambridge University Press, 2003.

[8] See a review on this topic, Luis Garicano and Luis Rayo, "Why Organizations Fail: Seven simple models and some cases", *Journal of Economic Literature*, vol. 54, no. 1, 2016, pp. 137–92.

Table 9-1: Information and Incentives in Different Policy Areas of the Health-care Regulation

Topics	Degree of Conflicting Interest	Information Asymmetry (between central and local)	Professional Expertise
Pharmaceutical sector	High	Low	High
Competition policy	High	Medium	High
Entry of the private sector	High	Medium	Medium
Social health insurance regulation	Medium	High	High
Medical malpractice disputes	High	Medium	High
Tobacco uses	High	Low	Low

Source: compiled by the author.

Table 9-1 lists the degree of information asymmetry and conflicting interest for the regulatory policies in the Chinese health-care system. Issues such as which pharmaceutical products to procure in public hospitals, what standard a new drug will be approved and how to settle a medical malpractice dispute are highly dependent on professional expertise; however, many compromised decisions have been made to take into consideration the conflict of interest between different government departments and different levels of government.

For competition policy enforcement, professional expertise is necessary. However, local conditions are highly relevant for the existence of market dominance. The entry of the private sector may have to take into account the conflict of interest, especially at the local level. The information requirement in this area is not very high.

Relevant information on social health insurance is highly decentralised and different localities have different coverage and benefits. Professional knowledge is critical in this context.

Resolving medical malpractice dispute needs high professional knowledge; the conflict of interest between different government departments at the local level is evident, given local officials' concern for social stability. Similarly, regulating tobacco uses may need to address the high conflict of interest given that the industry contributes a sizeable sum to the fiscal revenue.

Circumstantial evidence discussed in this book shows that some institutional arrangements in the Chinese regulatory system could be second best in dealing with the trade-off between the incentive and information structure. For example, to address the high degree of decentralisation of information such as different levels of local income, infrastructure and industrial structure, the local regulatory agency for social insurance has been given high authority by the upper level governments at the expense of economies of scale and scope.

In consequence, the capacity level may not be sufficient in these second best institutional arrangements. For example, local social insurers may not have strong bargaining power in their negotiations with hospitals given that high professional expertise is required to calculate risk and in making the arrangements of reimbursement.

However, in many cases, the institutional arrangement is suboptimal because of reasons other than the trade-off between incentives and information. For example, many institutional reforms fail because of the lack of political will or ineffective coordination among different government departments.[9] In some other cases, institutional reforms could not be implemented because they are not compatible with bureaucrats' interests or departmental interests.[10]

Another implication from Table 9-1 is that it is not necessary to have a unique institutional arrangement for decision-making right allocation given the different information and incentive structures. In the literature on business management, organisational forms indeed can be very different in different contexts.[11]

---

[9] See an example in Qian Jiwei and Mok Ka-Ho, "Dual Decentralization and 'Fragmented Authoritarianism' in Governance".

[10] Mario Gilli, Li Yuan and Qian Jiwei, "Logrolling under Fragmented Authoritarianism: Theory and evidence from China".

[11] Robert Simons, *Levers of Organization Design: How managers use accountability systems for greater performance and commitment*, Cambridge, Harvard Business Press, 2013.

To implement the institutional reforms, an alternative solution is to address the information and incentive trade-offs by taking advantage of the multi-dimensional aspects of the decision-making right. Given different degrees of conflicting interests and information asymmetry, according to the literature, the decision-making right can also be split into different dimensions to achieve a second best solution. For example, the division of decision-making right could be set based on formal and informal authority.[12] In some cases, the formal authority/decision-making right can be centralised and the informal authority/de facto authority can be delegated to lower division or decentralised. In other cases, the decision-making right can be divided into the right to set targets, the right to evaluate and the right to incentivise agents.[13] For example, in the case of environment regulation enforcement in China, the right to incentivise agents has been delegated (informally) to the city level while the right to set targets and evaluate has been centralised at the provincial level.[14]

Following this rationale and based on the multi-dimensional nature of the decision-making right, there can be multiple institutional arrangements to address the incentive and information trade-off. The solutions for the constraint of institutional arrangements are therefore not unique. Policy experimentation in this case may be helpful.[15]

---

[12] Philippe Aghion and Jean Tirole, "Formal and Real Authority in Organizations".

[13] Zhou Xueguang and Lian Hong, "Modes of Governance in the Chinese Bureaucracy: A 'control right' theory", *Journal of Sociological Research*, vol. 5, 2012, pp. 69–93.

[14] Zhou Xueguang and Lian Hong, "Modes of Governance in the Chinese Bureaucracy".

[15] See an example of this in another context in Qian Jiwei "Improving Policy Design and Capacity from Local Experiments: Equalization of public service in China's urban-rural integration pilot", *Public Administration and Development*, vol. 37, no. 3, 2017, pp. 51–64.

Index

Printed in the United States
By Bookmasters